Confidence Unleashed

Be the Unstoppable Hero of Your Own Heart

Laine D'Souza

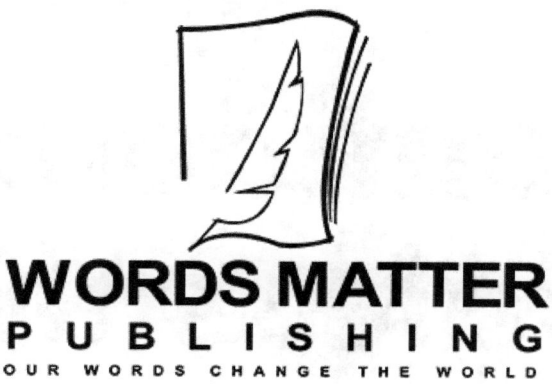

Words Matter Publishing
P.O. Box 1190
Decatur, IL 62525
www.wordsmatterpublishing.com

ISBN: 978-1-958000-76-2

Library of Congress Catalog Card Number: 2023946189

Dedication

To all the children of the universe, may you always know your worth. May you take action to become the humans you wish to be. May you always be grateful for the life you are 100% responsible for creating.

Table of Contents

To My Ever-Resilient Body,

I extend my heartfelt gratitude to you, my badass vessel, for your unwavering support throughout my incredible journey. You've cradled my two precious blessings, displaying an indomitable strength as you allowed me to carry them into this world. You've been my partner in joy, enabling me to dance, run, play, and boldly lift the weight of life's fiercest challenges.

In moments of weakness, you've stood tall, defiantly resisting the grip of sickness, bouncing back with remarkable resilience whenever I've faltered in my care. You've endured my demands without flinching, never wavering in your unyielding commitment to me. Even when I've taken you for granted, you've remained steadfast and true, radiating strength in the face of adversity.

My magnificent body, I thank you from the depths of my badass soul.

With boundless love and a fiery spirit,
Laine

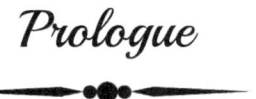

Prologue

You Versus You

> "You had the power all along, my dear."
> ~ *Glinda, Wizard of Oz*

Hey You,

Allow me to introduce myself—I am Laine D'Souza. Just a woman of forty-seven, who, like many, has traversed the winding roads of life, sometimes feeling adrift and inadequate. At the tender age of eight, I grappled with self-doubt, and the choices I made mirrored this inner turmoil. My life's journey has been a quest to uncover my gifts, share them, and liberate others from the shackles of self-doubt. To me, this is greatness: overcoming oneself.

GREATNESS IS OVERCOMING YOURSELF!

I don't wield credentials as a licensed therapist, doctor, or renowned expert. I don't stand as the best at anything, nor do I command vast speaking fees. I am simply a woman who once battled low self-esteem, and the consequences of my self-perception echoed in my choices. Yet, I've come to realize I'm not alone in this struggle. Many have forgotten their true selves, and I embarked on a journey to find mine.

I am just ME, and today, I stand proud of who I am and the person I work daily towards aspiring to become. It has taken forty-seven years—a treacherous journey filled with lessons, errors, failures, and too many wrong turns to lead me here. I can now place my hand over my heart and offer gratitude to all the women who paved the way. I refuse to compromise my values or seek approval from anyone but the reflection in my mirror. My self-opinion matters most.

As a certified personal trainer, indoor cycling instructor, certified CrossFit L1 coach, and yoga instructor, Gym Owner, I've had the privilege of training hundreds of women over the past twenty-five-plus years. Their stories have both touched and broken my heart. Hearing how they perceive their bodies, laden with self-loathing, shame, guilt, and unworthiness, mirrors the struggles I once faced. They, too, have suffered the self-inflicted wounds of believing they are not enough. Their bodies often bear the brunt of this inner turmoil. They despise their appearance, but through years of training women, I've come to understand—it's not about how they look but how they believe they look and how they feel about themselves.

Imagine if we could train our minds as we train our bodies, nurturing self-love just as we cultivate biceps. This would revolutionize the health and fitness industry. If these incredible women could see themselves through my eyes, recognizing their boundless potential, they could achieve anything. To me, that's the essence of coaching—unveiling someone's potential, equipping them with tools, and providing a safe, supportive environment where they can flourish.

I learned to see myself through the eyes of those who truly saw and believed in me. This allowed me to tap into my own gifts and offer value and results. After years of working with women, I know my feelings are not isolated. Thus, I felt compelled to use my voice, summoning the courage to reach out a helping hand to anyone who may be suffering.

I've penned this book with the hope of sharing my story and touching your life. It is a gift to you, to my inner child of ten, to my daughter, her daughter, and all those who can relate and yearn to conquer their inner battles. I aim to save you time and offer a roadmap. With practice, you can embark on daily rituals that will illuminate the path to self-discovery, allowing you to create not only yourself but the life you envision. I want you to recognize your immeasurable worth, and to understand that your past does not define you. You possess the power to heal and, in that healing, to foster the confidence to mold your dreams into reality.

I wrestled with profound self-esteem issues too. So, before we dive further into this journey, let's clarify what self-esteem truly means:

SELF-ES·TEEM
/SELFƏˈSTĒM/
NOUN

CONFIDENCE IN ONE'S OWN WORTH OR ABILITIES; SELF-RESPECT

These may appear as mere words, but they carry the potential to shape your life in ways both profound and transformative. A life without self-esteem can lead to paralysis, fear, and self-inflicted punishment, eroding your trust in yourself and obscuring your chosen path. I've walked this path, and I'm here to tell you—the gravity of living without self-esteem is too steep a cost. It's time to cultivate it.

I will unveil how I created it. I will elucidate how I nurtured it. I will share how I made it a daily practice. I will demonstrate that by embracing daily habits, you can craft your own happiness.

Now, let us continue. Practice, and embark on the journey of making yourself proud!

With All My Unwavering Love,
Laine
xo

Chapter One

---•◆•---

The Symphony of Resilience

"If you give a man a fish, you feed him for a day. If you teach a man to fish, you feed him for a lifetime."

~ Lao Tzu

In the heart of the relentless Urban Jungle of NYC, where dreams are forged and shattered by the minute, I embarked on a quest to redefine health. It's a symphony, an intricate dance of physical prowess, mental fortitude, and the audacity to soar. To me, 'Health' is more than a sterile definition; It's a kaleidoscope with many colors, shapes and dimensions of self discovery, courage, and an unyielding pursuit of excellence.

While the World Health Organization offers a noble description of health as complete physical, mental, and social well-being, I yearn for a definition that pulsates with vitality. Health is an art; it's the embodiment of resilience, the sacred ability to not just survive but thrive, body, mind, and spirit. A constant delicate changing balance, requiring shifting left, and right and is constantly ever vibrantly alive. Challenging you to be courageous enough to listen to your own body which is created with Devine intelligence in a world constantly enticing you to follow a trendy, doubt yourself and question a common sense attitude.

Imagine harnessing the miraculous power nestled within our beings, a divine force capable of regeneration and rebirth. It's the siren's call of possibility that urges us to recreate ourselves, to sculpt the very essence of who we long to be. This is the audacious spirit coursing through our veins.

Our journey commences with a passionate love affair, an unapologetic romance with the nurturing and healing of ourselves. Without our health, what remains?

As a youth, I reveled in the vibrancy of the tropics, a canvas painted with outdoor escapades, swimming pools, dance, and sports. Health, at that time, was a purely physical concept. Yet, the day my Olympic dreams slipped through my fingers, I learned that it transcended mere physicality. I lacked the mental tools, mentors, and guidance to navigate the treacherous waters of self-improvement. I faltered, and I quit. I let myself down and this was the slippery road that led to me having to climb and fight my way back to my true nature, my north star, my God-given blueprint.

If only I could journey back in time and whisper to my younger self,

"Failure is but a transient shadow, dear sweet girl. It does not define you. What defines you is your response, your resilience."

Alas, I allowed that setback to mold my identity, my choices, and my path.

To be the hardest worker in the room, I've discovered, is far more commendable than relying solely on the fleeting embrace of talent. I fell prey to the belief that I wasn't good enough, using it as armor against the specter of failure. This mindset dictated my choices, held me captive, and veiled my true potential. I was in agony, aware of my destined greatness yet imprisoned by self-doubt.

The Universe hadn't given up on me; it granted me a second chance to pursue my passion. I secured a spot in a prestigious dance college in London, despite lacking formal training or foundational skills. The dance committee recognized something unique in my freestyle and contemporary dance, and they believed in my potential. However, there was a condition: I had to improve my math grades to secure my college entry.

This requirement triggered my protective mechanisms and deep-seated beliefs about not being good enough. My self-doubt, the very thing that had held me back for so long, began to resurface. "I am dyslexic. Math and I just don't click," I reasoned.

To succeed in this endeavor, I realized that I had to become the hardest worker in the room. I had to be willing to risk giving my all and possibly falling short. The voices of doubt, excuses, and self-imposed limitations whispered to me, "Math is something your brain struggles with, causing stress, overthinking, and overwhelming thought patterns. It's not important; who needs more than basic arithmetic?" These voices urged me to stay small, to remain wounded, and to shy away from the spotlight.

I was not oblivious to this destructive pattern, yet it still manifested itself physically. My anxiety manifested as constant IBS (irritable bowel syndrome), food sensitivities, and allergies—an external reflection of my unprocessed emotions. This cycle continued, trapping me in the web of self-sabotage.

When I inevitably missed the math mark by a single point, I spiraled into a deep depression. I withdrew from social interactions and lost my sense of purpose. The voices of unworthiness grew louder, paralyzing me. Looking back, I wish I could travel back in time to coach my younger self, to impart the wisdom that talent and hard work are only small parts of greatness. The missing ingredient for true excellence lies within our minds—the choices we make in how we think, feel, and act in our lives.

Once more, we witness the profound connection between our thoughts and our mental well-being, which in turn affects our physical health. From my own childhood experiences, I've come to understand that health encompasses more than just physicality. Our mental state influences every aspect of our existence, from how we internalize and process experiences to our relationships with others and the world around us. Our thoughts and emotions play a pivotal role in shaping the outcomes of our circumstances and the trajectory of our lives.

In addition to our internal world, our external environment also molds our health, much like soil nutrients and sunlight nourish a blossoming flower. Our physical well-being reflects the external factors we encounter—our food and nutrition choices, our need for the "sunlight" of positivity, and the movement of our bodies and our resilience to heal.

It was during this dark period that I realized a vital truth: talent and hard work are mere puzzle pieces in the grand tapestry of greatness. The missing link is the mental game, the choices we make, the way we think, feel, and act. This insight laid the foundation for my future journey, the journey of becoming a stronger, more resilient human.

Health, I came to understand, transcends mere physicality. It encompasses our mental state, our emotional resilience, and our ability to connect with ourselves and the world around us. Our environment molds our health, just as nature shapes a flower's bloom. Our choices, our nutrition, our need for sunlight and movement—they all contribute to the masterpiece of our well-being.

Once, living in the heart of New York City, I fell seriously ill. A wise doctor noticed my narrow ear canals and attributed it to my adaptation to a water-centric childhood. Our bodies, he explained, are indeed clever, adapting to our early surroundings.

Exercise became my sanctuary, a refuge where I could nurture myself and conquer my inner demons. It was a form of moving meditation, a natural high that allowed me to transcend my limitations. It saved me during my darkest hours, providing an escape from my own thoughts.

Upon graduating, I embarked on an acting journey but faced crippling stage fright that forced me to abandon the spotlight. My path shifted again, leading me to become a personal trainer. This, I thought, was my safe haven, a place where I could excel without fear of inadequacy.

I encountered a diverse array of clients, each with their unique stories and struggles. I observed the profound impact of mindset on their journeys to health and happiness. Success was not solely determined by physical prowess but by the alignment of thoughts and actions.

Working within the fitness industry, I uncovered its dark underbelly, where appearances often trumped genuine well-being. I witnessed trainers promoting healthy lifestyles while indulging in fast food and even steroids. Corporate pressures to meet sales quotas tainted the noble goal of transforming lives.

The health and fitness industry, I realized, thrives on confusion, feeding the insecurities of its patrons. It's a multi-billion-dollar machine that preys on the vulnerable, promising quick fixes instead of love, true healing, and the individual.

Amidst these revelations, I discovered that emotional struggles are universal. We all battle the voices of self-doubt and insecurity. What sets us apart is our ability to amplify the voice that urges us to persist, to drown out the crippling whispers.

To those held captive by insecurity, I offer this: cherish that faint voice, even if it is but a whisper, for it holds the key to your liberation. Find a sanctuary, a passion, a place where that voice can grow stronger, a voice that says, 'You've got this!'

No matter if it is a mere whisper every 4th day, it just might be your wind, your guiding light, your mentor, or your inner divinity. Nurture it, for it's the catalyst for your transformation.

Healing, I discovered, is a journey toward self-acceptance. It's a process of making peace with past wounds, a process that doesn't erase the pain but reframes it into a source of strength. This healing journey unlocked my sense of emotional freedom, my inner peace, and my refusal to abandon myself.

The path to health is not one-size-fits-all; it's a unique journey for each of us. However, what unites us is the universal struggle against our inner demons and the choice to listen to the voice that encourages us to shine.

In a world flooded with confusing health information, the power lies in our hands. We must choose to empower ourselves, to navigate the labyrinth of choices, and to create our own path to well-being.

So, my fellow travelers on the road to health and fitness, I leave you with this thought:

"Learn to fall in Love with Taking Care of And Healing Yourself, without your Health what do you really have?"

Chapter Two

---•—◆—•---

Unlocking Your Inner Power: Embrace the Art of SWEAT

"Knowing is not enough; we must apply. Willing is not enough; we must do."

~ Bruce Lee

SWEAT = STOP WASTING ENERGY AND TIME

Let me begin by confessing that the daily ritual of exercise is far from easy for me. I struggle to find the motivation to start, often needing to push myself with affirmations and mantras like, "I am powerful!" The contrary voice in my head tends to be louder, whispering, "This is hard, ugh!" or "This hurts, ugh!" On those challenging days, my holy 'why' comes to the rescue.

I know, deep down, from personal experience, that exercise lifts a cloud from my being and allows me to be my best self. It's my daily practice, as essential as flossing my teeth. Those days when I battle with myself to start or conjure countless excuses not to move my body are fleeting and hold no significance in my daily agenda. I've established non-negotiable actions that truly matter to me because I refuse to be stuck in the same circumstances a year from now.

Learning to let go of thoughts, judgments, old beliefs, habits, and stories that shackle you is essential for progress. I've cultivated a practice of allowing that child-like voice within me to chatter without attaching myself to it. Initiating motion with my body, oddly enough, calms my central nervous system, making me feel safe. Soon, the workload dwindles, and I find myself basking in an endorphin cocktail of high gratitude. My central nervous system shifts from a fight-or-flight response to a serene state. Sweat, I've discovered, is akin to crying, a means of elimination, and I've chosen to sweat daily.

Making a commitment entails knowing that there will be days when you won't feel like it. Circumstances will arise, moods will shift, and distractions will beckon. However, the reward lies on the other side—the satisfaction of conquering your inner resistance, the natural chemical high, and the confidence boost when those skinny jeans fit just right. It's about creating peristaltic motion that flushes toxins from the inside out, enhancing mood, improving sleep, and staving off the specter of dementia that haunts my particular family history.

Despite being aware of the logical benefits and the miraculous healing power of exercise, it remains a formidable challenge, a path where you must earn your progress. You can't simply buy your way to fitness. It's an arena that teaches you how to navigate your inner dialogue when the pressure is on. Intentionally subjecting yourself to pressure builds grit, resilience, and a formidable mindset, preparing you for the unpredictable turns of life. Affirmations become your allies: "I am powerful. I've got this. Focus on squeezing your hips." I do it because, quite simply, I love the person I become after the battle, and I cherish the way I feel.

Back when I worked as a trainer in the bustling heart of New York City, one question reverberated more frequently than any other: "Why can't I lose weight?" People would approach me with a fixed goal in mind, often reduced to a number on the scale—125 pounds, for instance. Let's set something straight:

WHEN IT COMES TO NUMBERS, USE THEM FOR MEASUREMENT, NOT JUDGMENT!

GET OFF THE SCALE AND EMBRACE BODY COMPOSITION!

MUSCLE WILL SAVE YOUR LIFE!

Unless you're training for a specific weight category in a sport or competition, the number on the scale carries minimal significance. Many individuals may tip the scales at a mere 110 pounds but remain the unhealthiest, skinny-fat souls, burdened by high visceral fat—the very epitome of obesity by body fat percentage. Is that truly your goal? A mere number on the scale? Unlikely, when you utter a target weight, you're essentially envisioning a desired body aesthetic and attaching a numerical value to it. Instead, shift your focus to body fat percentage—the scale is but a rudimentary measure of health and fitness, an inept one at that. It reveals nothing about the actual progress being made. To be frank, the Body Mass Index (BMI) is an antiquated and inadequate measure that still inexplicably lingers in the medical realm.

Consider this scenario: You've shed fifteen inches in total, and lashed your body fat percentage by 7%, and yet the scale either remains immovable or, maddeningly, inches upward by three pounds. So, when tracking fitness achievements, banish the scale from your calculations if that's all it is to you, opt for better methods.

With that out of the way, let's focus on weight loss—or better yet, getting fit. One of the swiftest routes to shedding unwanted pounds is good old-fashioned running, swimming, and cycling. Cardio, or aerobic exercise, encompasses activities like running, rowing, cycling, and swimming. If you can't partake in one due to physical limitations, choose another that suits you. For me, power walking and running serve as moving meditations, offering mental solace and that coveted runner's high.

However, cardio isn't about the same monotonous routine day in and day out; variety is key. If running is your forte, try different techniques: a leisurely, extended jog one day, followed by a spirited Fartlek session (an enjoyable word to pronounce), a training technique used in running that means 'Speed Play' where you alternate between sprints and slow jogs often in an unstructured spontaneous manner. Next time, attempt a pace run—start slow, pick up speed in the middle, and ease into a cool-down at the end. Explore interval runs to hone your pace and consistency. Mix it up, keep it exciting, make it fun.

Keeping tabs on your progress is crucial to sustaining motivation. Observe how you feel after each session. Are you recuperating faster? Does that mile feel less daunting today? Adapting to your routines is equally important. Perhaps today you'll run, tomorrow you'll swim (an excellent choice), and the next day, you'll tackle a rowing workout. Keep it engaging and stay focused on your objectives.

Now, venture forth and make those pavements or tires scorch! Remember, your current condition is but the starting point, not the final destination. If you can only spare five minutes, then do five minutes, but do it every day! It might involve running or cycling to your favorite song. The next time, aim for six or more minutes. Play your inspirational tune twice. The key is to initiate action. Cultivate happiness by appreciating what you can do today, building upon it day by day.

Whether you lose or gain weight, remember that the numbers can't gauge your efforts or victories. They can't reveal your progress or the invaluable lessons you've learned. They can't measure your growth or your self-earned accomplishments. Instead, consider photographs as a superior visual guide.

At the end of the day, they are mere numbers—best employed for measurements and tracking, not for judgments.

Within the boundless wave of human existence, we find ourselves entwined with a force as ancient as the Earth itself: the power of sweat. As we've journeyed through these pages, you've glimpsed the profound impact of this elixir; how it sculpts not just our bodies but our destinies, how it transforms not just our skin but our souls. Sweat, my fellow seekers of greatness, is the ink with which we write our stories of triumph. It's the universal currency of effort, the elixir of tenacity, and the catalyst of boundless potential.

In your every drop of perspiration, you've distilled determination. In each bead that glistens on your brow, you've embodied resilience. Remember, when you embrace the sweat, you embrace the relentless pursuit of excellence. The path to self-mastery, to liberation from the constraints of doubt, begins with a single drop, then a river, then an ocean of your own sweat equity.

As you embark on your journey, let this truth be your compass: within every pour of sweat lies the promise of transformation. It's not just about the physical benefits, though they are plentiful. It's about the metamorphosis of the spirit, the forging of an indomitable will, and the emergence of a warrior unafraid to chase their dreams.

So, my sweat enthusiasts, remember to revel in the sheen of your efforts, embrace the discomfort as the birthplace of your strength, and cherish every drop as the nectar of your ascent. For in the world of sweat, champions are crafted, dreams are realized, and limits cease to exist.

Go forth and conquer, armed with the knowledge that within your sweat, you hold the keys to your own radiant destiny. May you continue to sweat with purpose, and may every drop propel you closer to the extraordinary life you were meant to lead!

Chapter Three

---•●•---

Forged in Fire: The Unbreakable Spirit of Self-Transformation

"You can go to the gym, drink your water and take your vitamins but if you don't deal with the shit going on in your head and heart, you're still going to be unhealthy."

~ Lewis Howes

Our bodies are marvels of regeneration and healing. True fitness encompasses more than just physical prowess. It encompasses your capacity to recover from stress, trauma, and life's vicissitudes. This recovery doesn't exclusively pertain to exercise; it extends to emotional resilience, environmental challenges, and overcoming the odds—truly thriving, not merely surviving.

WHAT IS FITNESS?

"The condition of being physically fit and healthy."

From an athlete's perspective, physical fitness extends beyond just the body's ability to recuperate. It's about pushing your heart rate to its limits and then witnessing how quickly you can return to equilibrium. You see, fitness transcends physical recovery alone.

For me, exercise is about more than just aesthetics. It's about feeling capable and trusting my body. Could I outrun someone or something if the situation arose? The answer is an unequivocal yes. Confidence courses through me, in knowing I can rise to any challenge in life.

In the quest for fitness, it's not just about numbers on a scale or the aesthetics of your physique; it's about the strength, speed, and unwavering belief in yourself that emerges from the crucible of exercise. Fitness is a lifelong journey, one that involves maximizing your potential as a human being. Some may criticize your dedication to lifting weights or paying attention to your diet, but ultimately, it's your life, and you must live it in your body.

It's wonderful to fit into those skinny jeans and feel confident in your own skin, but the true beauty lies in knowing that you possess the strength and capability to handle challenging situations. Fitness isn't just about appearances; it's about building resilience and belief in your own body, allowing you to run after your kids or chase down a thief who swiped your wallet.

Exercise, for me, represents more than a desire to look good— it's about knowing that I can trust my body when I need it most. Whether it's outrunning a threat or embracing the confidence that comes with endurance, it's about mastering the art of doing difficult things.

During my school years, I was often the last one picked for teams in gym class. I couldn't run without gasping for air, and my legs ached from even the shortest sprints. It was a humbling experience that tested my perseverance. Yet, in those moments of vulnerability, I discovered my own resilience. It wasn't about winning races or impressing others; it was about pushing past my limits and surprising myself with what I could achieve.

In my formative years, school was an uphill battle. As a dyslexic student, I felt insecure about my intellectual abilities. I was teased for struggling with reading aloud and relegated to special math and English classes. While others played basketball, I wrestled with grammar. Reading comprehension seemed an insurmountable obstacle. Rather than excel academically, I used my energy to excel physically in sports, where I found solace and trust in my abilities. When performing well in sports occasionally failed me, exercise remained my sanctuary.

So, as you embark on your fitness journey, remember that it's okay to be vulnerable. It's okay to struggle, to gasp for breath, and to feel the burn in your muscles. Embrace that vulnerability, for it's the crucible in which strength and resilience are forged. It's the place where you'll discover the power of your own body and the depth of your determination.

In the world of fitness, vulnerability is not a weakness; it's a badge of honor. It's a testament to your courage and your willingness to push through discomfort in pursuit of your goals. So, sweat it out, embrace the struggle, and know that with every drop of sweat, you're not just transforming your body; you're unveiling a power that resides within you.

As you continue this journey, remember that the most beautiful aspect of fitness is not the sculpted physique you'll achieve, but the unwavering belief in yourself that will carry you through life's challenges. So, keep sweating, keep pushing, and keep believing in your own strength.

I aspired to be someone who manifested my dreams, ideas, and thoughts—a force of nature whose energy was contagious. I was driven to fulfill my promises, to be a person whose determination overpowered the fear of thinking I couldn't. Embracing discomfort and sacrifice became my modus operandi, fueled by my unwavering desire to attain my goals.

WHAT IF WE COULD SHIFT OUR PERCEPTION OF EXERCISE, RECOGNIZING IT AS A DIVINE GIFT?

It fortifies our immunity. While the health industry is focused on curative medicine, striving to find remedies for existing ailments, fitness epitomizes preventive medicine—a robust defense against sickness and the key to security. We must defend ourselves, not just against physical exertion but emotional tests and mental pitfalls. It's about thriving, not merely surviving. Exercise, for me, extends beyond mere aesthetics; it's about trusting myself and my body to withstand the rigors of life.

Yet, from these uncertain beginnings, I unearthed a resilient spirit. I channeled my energies into the physical realm, finding solace and trust in sports. When, occasionally, even sports betrayed me, I felt adrift, but I always had the sanctuary of exercise. I longed for the elation of self-approval, the embrace of self-love, and the transcendence into a realm where my vibrant energy could ignite the world. I aspired to be the embodiment of my promises, the kind of person whose determination blazed so fiercely that when I declared my intentions, others had a choice: join my journey or step aside. My desire to achieve greatness outweighed any fear that sought to hold me back.

I learned to welcome the discomfort and sacrifices on the path to my desires. I embraced the pain, knowing it was the crucible in which I would create my dreams, beliefs, and thoughts into reality. The pain was the price of progress, a small toll I gladly paid to avoid being enslaved by old habits and doubts.

Why do I train? Not for external accolades or to prove anything to others. I train to evoke a sense of pride and accomplishment within myself, to conquer the excuses that threaten to undermine my resolve.

Imagine if we reframed exercise as a divine gift, a fortification of our bodies. While the health industry focuses on curing ailments, fitness is the prophylactic safeguard that prevents the onset of illness. I train for life itself, making it an integral part of my daily routine, much like brushing my teeth or nourishing my body. Just as I maintain financial reserves, I believe in maintaining a physical reserve—a reserve of health, strength, and immunity. I aim to be prepared for the unexpected, to face sickness or surgery with a body primed for recovery. As I age, I don't wish to shrink my world; I want to expand it. My body is a vessel, and I intend to keep it seaworthy for the voyage ahead.

I don't train for appearance alone. I train for the sensation, the feeling of strength, capability, and self-assuredness. When you show up consistently and subject your body to stress, it will adapt and evolve naturally to meet the challenge, sculpting itself in the process. Too often, we fixate on the outcome, overlooking the profound impact of the journey itself.

Fitness isn't a trend or a passing fad; it's a lifelong commitment to maximizing human potential. Critics may scoff at my dedication to exercise and my meticulous dietary choices, but I don't live for their approval. I live for myself and my experience in this body. Why wouldn't I strive to feel my best?

Fitting into skinny jeans or confidently donning a bikini is undeniably satisfying, but the true joy comes from knowing that I possess the strength and resilience to tackle life's unexpected challenges. My training isn't just about physical prowess; it's about cultivating a mindset that empowers me to overcome any obstacle.

Remember the question: "What if no one is coming to save you?" I asked myself if I could, and my resounding answer was yes. I want to be self-reliant, capable of pulling myself up in the face of adversity. It all begins with the commitment to doing hard things and training ourselves for life's unexpected demands.

My training partner, a petite kickboxer, taught me a powerful lesson. She faced a life-threatening situation, but her physical conditioning allowed her to escape from danger. In moments of heightened adrenaline and life-or-death urgency, she knew she could rely on herself.

Fitness is more than just the improvement of your body; it's about enhancing your mind and spirit. It's about understanding that the true measure of health and fitness lies in our ability to thrive outside the gym, adapt to life's challenges, and succeed in our endeavors.

I learned this lesson through a traumatic experience that, in retrospect, was a gift. It taught me that fitness is a key to self-confidence, accomplishment, and pride. These qualities cannot be bestowed; they must be earned through dedication and consistency.

So, I encourage you to take action. Make movement a part of your daily life, cultivating a sense of pride and emotional security. Incorporating both cardiovascular exercise and resistance training into your fitness routine, with a minimum frequency of at least twice a week for each, varying in duration and intensity is essential for maintaining overall health. This comprehensive approach promotes cardiovascular health by enhancing your heart's efficiency and capacity while reducing the risk of chronic diseases, while also strengthening your muscles and bones, which is crucial for maintaining posture, strength, and mobility and preventing age-related decline. Build a routine that makes you feel proud of yourself, knowing that happiness isn't something you wait for; it's something you create. Trust yourself to be the architect of your own happiness and success.

Take action, find a fitness regimen that excites you, and commit to it daily. Know yourself, understand your triggers, and adapt your routine to suit your life. By creating a daily life that fills you with pride and emotional security, you'll find the confidence and trust in yourself to create your own happiness, rather than relying on others or external circumstances to do so.

As I pondered my role in class, struggling to keep up with my peers, I realized I had to forge my path to success. I had to navigate a world that often told me I wasn't good enough. I channeled my energy into physical pursuits and sports. When I was let down, exercise remained my constant.

Today, I challenge my old mindset. I'm here, bearing my mistakes and failures for judgment. Writing this book, I'm no longer seeking approval, for my conversations are between me and my creator. 'His' opinion and mine are the only ones that matter. This journey is a testimony to gratitude, as it unfolds into lessons—often costly—that reveal the gem, the gift, the healing.

"I'm not sure I can do it; people will say it's not grounded in this or that, and blah, blah, blah. But if it reaches and touches someone's heart and moves them into action, then this book and its message have served their purpose. I got over myself to shine a light on someone else. I cannot die with my song, lesson, and voice left unsung. If I don't try, there's no dignity in that."

So, here is your call to action:

CREATE SPACE!

Make time in your life for movement today. Establish a daily routine where small habits accumulate, fostering self-confidence, pride, and a sense of accomplishment. These are virtues you must earn by consistently showing up; they cannot be bestowed, bought, or sold. Join my community and overcome yourself every day.

TAKE ACTION!

Find a trainer, a class, an app, or a training partner, and consider signing up for a competition. Discover something that excites you about moving your body regularly, then carve out a specific time each day to commit to it as a non-negotiable part of your daily routine.

KNOW THYSELF!

Part of achieving success is recognizing your mindset, understanding your body, and identifying triggers. If evenings tend to become chaotic with familial responsibilities or fatigue, or if work prolongs your day, shift your workout to the morning. If you're not a morning person, set an alarm and dedicate your mornings to your well-being. If you ever experience overwhelming sensations without a logical explanation, take a few moments to sit with that discomfort, breathe deeply, and remind yourself that you are safe and loved.

By molding your daily life into a tapestry of pride, emotional safety, and physical well-being, you'll draw closer to nurturing an inner sense of trust and self-confidence. Don't wait for happiness or someone else to hand it to you; create it yourself.

In the early days of my New York City adventure, my apartment building in the East Village harbored a gym in its basement—a haven for old-school bodybuilders. These individuals, masters of sculpting their physiques through nutrition and training, mesmerized me. I observed as they transformed their bodies into unique shapes, each the embodiment of their dedication.

One woman, in particular, undertook an arduous journey in preparation for a bodybuilding show. She diligently adhered to a strict diet, tracking every macronutrient down to the last gram. As the show date drew near, her obsession with precision escalated. She became withdrawn, moody, and fixated on her diet. Her skin erupted with breakouts, and she lost her menstrual cycle due to extreme dietary restrictions. On the day of the show, she dehydrated herself to enhance vascularity, leading to a painful urinary tract infection. She could barely summon the strength to perform, and as soon as she stepped off stage, she found herself in the emergency room, attached to IVs. The spectacle was both fascinating and bewildering—a sport that demanded so much dedication yet led to the brink of peril due to body image and dietary obsessions, all hanging on the eye of a subjective judge.

People often asked if I, too, was a bodybuilder. I consistently declined, unwilling to cede power to a judge's subjective assessment of my body's symmetry or muscularity. I refused to be a participant in such a capricious sport, having witnessed the turmoil, and downward spiral so many women experienced—predominantly linked to their body image and food-related issues. Instead, I gravitated towards powerlifting competitions, where your success hinges on your ability to lift, not a judge's assessment of your physical appearance. This sport allowed me to seize control of my destiny and craft my own happiness.

If only I could impart one life principle to my younger self at sixteen, it would be that of a growth mindset. I wish I had known that my talents and abilities could be cultivated through dedication, hard work, and perseverance. A growth mindset shuns feelings of inadequacy and invites challenges with open arms. There's no such thing as failure; every experience serves as a stepping stone to greater growth. The fundamental belief is that your basic qualities are things you can nurture through effort, empowering you to own your choices and mindsets. My life could have taken a different trajectory if I had been introduced to the concept of a growth mindset—a world of innate talents waiting to flourish through preparation and hard work.

As you continue this journey, remember that the most beautiful aspect of fitness is not the sculpted physique you'll achieve, but the unwavering belief in yourself that will carry you through life's challenges. So, keep sweating, keep pushing, and keep believing in your own strength. As slowly you will begin to surprise yourself, you've got this.

Chapter Four

Puberty in My Feet, Curves in My Head: Cultivating Womb Safe

"A healthy mind has an easier breath."

~ Lyza Sahertian

Keep your head and feet in the same place. You might have heard this concept before. It's the essence of learning to keep your mind where your body is, cultivating and rediscovering what it means to feel truly safe within yourself.

When we react excessively and blow things out of proportion, our minds are signaling to our bodies that we are not safe; it's a call to attack, defend, or run. This reaction is deeply rooted in our body's memory and a trauma response. To address this, we need to delve into somatic healing, creating, and nurturing a sense of "womb safety" within ourselves when triggered by early childhood memories, adolescent betrayals, or moments when we felt deeply vulnerable:

"I'm not safe! I'm not enough! I'm going to be left! I'm not lovable. I'm alone! I'm not loved!"

Teaching your body that you are indeed safe is a matter of taming your nervous system, rather than relying solely on cerebral understanding. In these moments, rational thinking often falls short, and meditation alone won't suffice. It is essential to have effective tools at your disposal and self-awareness to practice them.

Learning to be and how to be present in the moment. When you feel that you're being taken advantage of or that you're under attack, it's essential to acknowledge the sensations bubbling up within you. You see, during these times, our minds can become overwhelmed with worries about the future, fears, doubts, and negative thoughts rooted in past experiences. In these moments, grounding yourself, using your breath, and becoming present are vital.

Our task is to teach our bodies, to work with our bodies, to rewire them, and to redefine what it means to feel safe and secure within ourselves. This process enables us to respond to present circumstances without reacting based on past experiences. By achieving this, we can be in relationships with others while maintaining a deep connection with ourselves, free from the disruptive influence of unresolved emotional triggers.

Once our nervous system is regulated, we gain the ability to distinguish between our emotions and those of others. We free ourselves from the unconscious patterns formed by our wounded inner child, which often lead to jealousy, insecurity, and fear. It all comes back to working with body memory and recognizing, in those critical moments, that we are indeed safe. This is the time to breathe into your feet and reassure your brain that you are here and now, and it's okay to let go of past fears. These moments present opportunities for self-nurturing, self-care, and indulging in activities that bring joy and fulfillment.

Learning to conquer insecurities starts with accepting where you are and making improvements toward where you want to be.

Forgive yourself for past mistakes, understanding that you did the best you could with the knowledge and resources you had at those moments. Without those lessons, you wouldn't be the person you are today. Now that you know better, you can do better.

Are you somewhere physically, yet your mind wanders to your grocery list, tomorrow's lunchbox packing, or replay conversations, betrayals, mistakes, or negative self-talk? Do you find it challenging to stop overthinking, get out of your head, and fully immerse yourself in the present moment? These are signs that the traumas you've endured are stored within you, impacting your daily life, influencing your thoughts and behaviors, and creating chaos.

Consider this: there are brain scans that depict brains exposed to trauma and 'normal' brains. Traumatized brains appear muddled and disorganized, while a 'normal' brain shows clear distinctions in each quadrant. Imagine walking through life with a brain that processes information like a milkshake, resulting in scrambled thoughts and difficulties in communication and understanding reality not a reality through your sense tainted from trauma. Many of us share this reality, grappling with unresolved trauma, which leads to chaos becoming the norm. Unless we actively seek the right healing, this distorted reality governs our lives and relationships.

It's essential to understand that trauma responses manifest differently for each person. However, a wise friend once taught me a valuable life principle based on AA principles:

"If it's hysterical (excessive, disproportionate), it's historical (rooted in past triggers)."

When faced with emotional reactions that seem overreactive or irrational, we can recognize them as echoes of past wounds. This awareness allows us to pause, reclaim our power, and acknowledge that we are experiencing body memory, even when we are safe in the present moment. It's an opportunity to breathe into our feet and reassure our minds that we are here, safe, and capable of managing these emotions.

In the depths of my soul, there existed a self-loathing that defied the love and support of my extraordinary family. Their unwavering care and encouragement should have been my foundation, but the relentless insecurities that gripped me were a shadow I couldn't escape. Dyslexia, the specter that haunted my educational journey, made the mere act of writing this book a venture beyond the wildest dreams of my former self. I recognize the message I carry, and I extend an olive branch to the grammar gatekeepers out there, urging them to embrace compassion over criticism as they listen to the message, not just scrutinize the messenger.

My schooling days were a labyrinth of challenges. I became a master of disguise, concealing the fact that numbers danced before my eyes and words played tricks on me. It took me twice as long as my peers to grasp the simplest concepts, to decipher the cryptic language of letters and sentences. While my classmates reveled in spirited games of basketball during recess, I languished in the isolation of special education classes, subjected to the ridicule of those who called us 'dummies.' The shame was inescapable, and it marked the genesis of my silent struggle, a struggle that would shadow my every step.

The well-intentioned 'help' I received had an unintended consequence. It taught me how to shut down, to withdraw into myself, to overcompensate, and pretend to be someone I wasn't, all in a desperate attempt to fit in. A dyslexic clinic and its array of treatments, even colored glasses that could have offered solace, became symbols of my longing for normalcy. I yearned to shed my 'owl face' and the taunts that followed, believing them to be echoes of my inadequacy. My slow reading and mispronounced words became a part of my identity, an identity steeped in the conviction that I wasn't smart enough.

At a tender age, I discovered the art of self-abandonment, a survival tactic to navigate a world that seemed intent on highlighting my deficits. In this self-neglect, I found the means to endure, to manipulate the system, and to provide people with the façade they sought. People-pleasing became my armor, shielding me from a world that seemed too cruel to accept the real me. Through avoidance and concealment, I managed to progress through school without truly comprehending or learning, evading the essentials like multiplication tables. The suppression of my voice, a voice stifled by laughter and mockery, created a dissonance between my outer silence and the tumultuous cacophony of my inner turmoil.

This is how I felt about what unfolded—I denied my emotions, rejected the existence of any problem, and dismissed the reality of my struggles. I had unearthed a superpower—the ability to be physically present while mentally escaping. I had checked out a skill so finely honed that it allowed me to traverse between the realms of left and right brain, a coping mechanism that enabled survival.

No one imparts the wisdom of navigating the transformations our bodies undergo, be it puberty, menopause, or any life-altering changes. The silence persists, shrouding our experiences, and leaving us unprepared for the uninvited gazes, the sudden disregard, or the internal battle with aging. It's time to expand our horizons, celebrate every number as a testament to our victories, and cherish the wisdom that comes with age, rather than retreat into shame.

As puberty swept through our lives, boys in my class initiated a sinister game of unwarranted advances. Flicked bra straps soon escalated into distressing encounters, where we felt cornered and violated against the unforgiving lockers. In my silence, I languished, trapped in a prison of self-loathing, unable to articulate my pain or fear. This pattern of self-betrayal and the inability to find my voice defined my existence. I had abandoned myself for the sake of acceptance, a silent witness to my own suffering.

The consequences of unaddressed trauma are insidious. It cloaks itself as a distant dream, and denial becomes its ally. We question whether it happened at all, and our minds detach from the body to escape the torment. Survival, it seems, hinges on refusing to acknowledge the truth. Yet, when we evade our demons, they seep into every crevice of our lives, a silent scream that others can discern behind our façade of outward confidence and masked insecurity.

I deeply resonate with the lotus flower, a symbol of transformation. "No mud, no lotus" perfectly encapsulates the idea that our transformative journey begins from the inside out. We must make peace with the darkness beneath the surface, where our fears, sadness, and anger reside. By acknowledging these emotions, we become objective observers of the present moment, shedding light on our inner world. This shift from primal fear to an evolved perspective allows us to experience, learn from, and grow through challenging emotions.

How do we achieve this presence? Contrary to traditional meditation, which often involves sitting still, I choose to move. Instead of checking out, I check in. I incorporate physical activity into my daily routine, such as running or weightlifting, to ground myself in the present moment. Exercise serves as my moving meditation, a way to be fully present in my body and mind.

Exercise is not about chasing after six-pack abs or societal beauty standards; it's about earning a feeling that cannot be bought. Exercise is breath work. Exercise plays a pivotal role in cultivating good movement patterns for posture and longevity, as it promotes neuromuscular coordination, enhances joint stability, and reinforces the structural integrity of our musculoskeletal system, thereby preventing postural imbalances, discomfort, and age-related issues, ensuring a healthier and more functional body in the long term. Focusing on good movement patterns is crucial beyond just fitting into your skinny jeans or rocking a six-pack because it incorporates longevity. It's about embracing discipline, doing hard things consistently, and experiencing the chemical rush of endorphins, serotonin, and dopamine—the body's natural medicine. For me, exercise is about taking control of my life and nurturing my body, mind, and spirit.

Resistance training is a fundamental aspect of reaching your goals efficiently. It involves movements that create resistance, such as weightlifting or resistance band exercises. The primary goal is to move weight, which helps increase bone density, maintain, or build muscle, and extend calorie burn long after the workout ends.

Let's address a common misconception: the fear of women becoming 'bulky' through resistance training. Let's stop this narrative in its tracks! Unless you possess the rare genetic predisposition to produce excessive testosterone and consume chicken breasts by the dozen, you needn't worry about gaining excessive muscle mass. The 'bulky' notion is a myth perpetuated by misunderstanding. The women who exhibit strong, muscular physiques did not simply stumble upon them; they meticulously dedicated themselves to years of weight training. They tailored their nutrition to support muscle growth, abiding by strict plans. They honed their discipline and commitment to pure bodybuilding movements, working within specific rep and set ranges to foster muscle hypertrophy. The misconception that weights make women 'bulky' is a disservice to the incredible dedication required to achieve such a physique, a result of careful planning and unyielding discipline. This common misconception that resistance training will make women bulky like men, must be stopped. This couldn't be further from the truth. Women generally lack the genetic hormonal predisposition and nutritional regimen required to achieve a "bulky" appearance. Building substantial muscle mass is a dedicated, intentional, and long-term endeavor that goes beyond lifting weights casually. Moreover, resistance training doesn't just shape the body; it strengthens the mind and deepens the connection between body and mind.

I encourage you to mix up your resistance training routine. Some days focus on movements with moderate weight and higher repetitions, while other days challenge yourself with heavier weights and lower repetitions. Consistency and variety are key to building a strong, healthy mind and body.

Exercise isn't merely about looking good; it's about feeling your best, expanding your life, and celebrating every number, whether high or low, as a victory. Age should be a celebration of wisdom and life lessons, not a source of shame or limitation.

Born in Hong Kong to an English mother and an Indian-Portuguese father, I often felt like I didn't belong anywhere. Regardless of my racial background, my inner feelings of isolation persisted. My life's journey has been about discovering my dreams, talents, and gifts while healing myself and empowering women to realize their worth and transcend their pasts. One of my gifts is the ability to see possibilities in people and things before they see them in themselves.

Within my core, there exists an unwavering determination, an unyielding spirit that thrives on embracing life's most formidable challenges. I'm known for my stubbornness, a relentless drive to conquer the seemingly insurmountable, for I've always believed that true growth and answers lie on the other side of adversity. Take, for instance, my irrational fear of public speaking, a fear at odds with my burning desire to become an actress. In a twist of fate, I subconsciously, and later consciously, sought out situations that ignited this fear within me, for it was only by confronting these demons that I could break free from their suffocating grip. I refused to remain a prisoner in my own life, suffocated by the voices that threatened to paralyze my journey toward self-realization.

The journey of healing took many forms for me, as I grappled with a profound sense of brokenness. I was open to every conceivable remedy, eager to unravel the complexities of my emotional turbulence. I yearned to transcend the shackles of reactivity that bound me, to master my emotions and quell the relentless anxiety that had held me hostage for far too long. My quest led me on a worldwide pilgrimage, seeking solace and enlightenment in a multitude of practices and philosophies. From deep-breathing exercises to the soothing embrace of yoga, from the enigmatic shadows of esoteric schools to the mysteries of Reiki, I delved into any avenue that offered the hope of healing my perceived wounds. I carried a heavy burden, convinced that something was fundamentally wrong within me, that salvation lay beyond my reach, held by external forces waiting to mend, forgive, and heal me. My search was external, driven by the relentless desire to be "fixed."

Raised in the Catholic faith, I had an unshakable connection to a divine creator, a sense of profound protection that cloaked me. Despite my skepticism of organized religion, I yearned to find meaning and belonging in spiritual practices. Yoga, meditation, shamanism, Buddhism, and even Mormonism, I explored them all in my desperate quest to escape the pervasive unease that haunted me. I sought refuge anywhere I could, hoping to find acceptance and silence the disquiet that plagued me.

As Rumi so eloquently stated, "Your task is not to seek for love, but merely to seek and find all the barriers within yourself that you built against it."

This season of my life taught me a vital life lesson—the only way out is to summon the courage to confront the past, to reconcile my mind and my heart in the present. It was a wise friend, a proponent of AA principles, who illuminated a path to understanding my reactive tendencies. Whenever I found myself on the precipice of an overly emotional response, teetering on the edge of hysteria, I realized that the emotion was always rooted in history, a relic of old wounds echoing through time. Recognizing these emotional landmines became my lifeline, a signal to pause, self-reflect, and unearth the unresolved traumas that lay beneath. Rather than react impulsively, I learned to respond consciously, regaining my power and agency in moments of emotional turbulence. This practice of checking in, rather than checking out, transformed my life and allowed me to escape the cycle of trauma.

Learning to sit with the discomfort, to confront the emotions I once sought to evade at any cost, became a pivotal lesson in my journey. It was the journey from denial to acceptance, from self-judgment to self-compassion, and from resistance to surrender. The path to healing required acknowledging the darkness lurking beneath the lotus, a journey that began with awareness. Much like cleaning a room in the dark, we must first illuminate our thoughts before we can transform them. Our thoughts are the rooms of our minds, and we must turn on the lights to tidy them. I no longer denied these emotions, nor did I attempt to change them; I simply acknowledged their presence. This awareness propelled me from the primal, fear-driven part of my brain to a more evolved state. It was the first step in cleaning my inner sanctuary, the step that allowed me to sit with the discomfort, breathe through it, and ultimately to transcend it. The way out, as it turns out, is through.

The lotus flower is special place to me, a symbol of beauty born from the muddiest waters. It encapsulates the essence of our transformative journey, an exploration that begins inside and radiates outward. The key lies in observing the darkness beneath the surface, in making peace with the murky depths that hold us captive. The process begins with awareness, for we can only change our thoughts once we recognize them. Just as a cluttered room cannot be cleaned in darkness, our thoughts require the light of awareness. When we honestly confront our emotions, we open the door to self-compassion, the space where growth and learning can flourish.

How do I stay present? I move. I run, I lift weights, and I simply engage with my body and surroundings. I check in, not out. I find solace in the rhythm of my breath during a round of sun salutations, grounding my feet and anchoring my mind to the present. For me, exercise is a moving meditation, a daily ritual that provides a sense of accomplishment, discipline, and an irreplaceable feeling that cannot be bought. It's about pursuing inner peace, embracing gratitude for the privilege of movement, and savoring the natural medicine of endorphins—gifts from a benevolent universe.

Resistance training is my conduit to self-discovery and transformation. It goes beyond the pursuit of physical aesthetics; it's about empowering my mind and body to surmount obstacles. Resistance training encompasses weightlifting, band exercises, and any movement that introduces resistance into each motion. Whether I'm performing push-ups, air squats, or lifting barbells, it's about moving against resistance to bolster bone density, preserve or build muscle, and engage in calorie-burning exercises that endure long after the workout ends.

Exercise, despite my initial reluctance and good intentions, became my compass, pointing me steadfastly north. It taught me not to abandon myself, to embrace discipline, and to persevere through tough times without seeking instant gratification. It illuminated the profound interconnectedness of mind, body, and spirit, fostering a profound realization—that health is not merely a physical endeavor; it encompasses the totality of our being. This is why I'm so impassioned about helping others feel their best, for I've witnessed firsthand the transformative power of nurturing one's physical and emotional well-being. It's not solely about looking good; it's about feeling your best, and sometimes, it's about changing your entire life in the process.

In overcoming our insecurities, we must first accept where we are and commit to improving ourselves. Forgiveness for past mistakes is paramount, recognizing that we did the best we could with the tools we had at the time. These lessons shaped us into who we are today, and now, armed with knowledge and self-compassion, we can strive for better. Remember, the journey to a better self begins with understanding, acceptance, and the unwavering commitment to being the best version of ourselves.

Chapter Five

---•◦•---

Rescued by Fitness: How College Became My Crucible of Transformation

"Knowing is not enough, we must apply. Willing is not enough, we must do."

~ Bruce Lee

Fitness has many faces. For me, it wasn't about striving for a perfect physique. Instead, it became a lifeline, a savior that I stumbled upon during my college years.

Growing up, I was fortunate to have an athletic dad. He instilled in us not the pursuit of a certain look, but the joy of movement itself. Our family time was spent bonding through sports, and it left a profound imprint on me.

However, it wasn't until I ventured into college that fitness took on a new significance. I was an athlete, with dreams that reached as far as Olympic trials. Sadly, I fell short, and the rejection felt personal. I internalized it, letting it gnaw at my sense of self. Looking back, I ache for that young woman who simply needed to work on her weaknesses, learn tenacity, and emerge stronger from the next trials.

College brought its own set of challenges, including a painful breakup that left me adrift. I abandoned not only my relationship but also my beliefs and my very sense of self. It was paralyzing. At the time, I was grappling with IBS to such an extent that my weight plummeted to a dangerous 85 pounds. I was a fragile shadow of myself, mentally and physically. I was lost and scared.

Yet, amid this turmoil, an unexpected angel arrived in my life. My socially awkward roommate decided, without consulting me, to bring home an old, smelly dog, a chocolate lab with a grey beard with behavioral issues! I resisted, but soon I realized that this dog, named Coco, would become my lifeline.

At that point, I could barely muster the strength to get out of bed, but Coco's attachment to me became my motivation. I had a reason to rise each day—not for myself, but for her. It marked the beginning of a co-dependence that saved me at the time, although later, I would learn the importance of letting go of such behaviors once their protective purpose had served its time.

Coco introduced me to running, an activity I never truly loved in terms of timing or distance. But I ran for Coco. It was the one thing that reassured me that everything would eventually be alright. Running silenced my overactive mind, quelled the nervousness in my stomach, and stilled my shaking limbs. For that precious hour, it allowed me to simply be, to inhabit my body fully. It was my therapy, my sanctuary, the respite that kept me moving forward when everything else seemed impossible.

I remember running to the top of hills in the heart of Wales, with America on one horizon and Ireland on the other. Those moments allowed me to dream big, to believe, even if just for a minute, that everything would be okay. It felt like the universe was pushing me forward, as though God's hands were on my back, guiding me when I couldn't do it for myself.

In the world of fitness, self-kindness is a vital element. Be gentle with your words, your thoughts, and your actions. Trust the process, knowing that each moment contributes to your growth and higher self.

Sharing the gift of exercise with others has been one of my true calling. It connected me with my creator, and ironically, one of my purposes in life taught me forgiveness. It reminded me that I am a Child of the Universe, regardless of circumstances. Fitness became my moving meditation.

It's not just about aesthetics; fitness taught me discipline, consistency, and the power of delayed gratification. It showed me that health encompasses mind, body, and spirit. I'm passionate about helping people feel their best because it's not solely about looking good; it's about feeling your best. Sometimes, it's about changing or saving your entire life.

Resilience is another gift I gleaned from my fitness journey. For me, resilience means finding meaning within failures, losses, and heartbreaks, as well as celebrating successes. I've learned to bounce back quickly from difficulties, much like the intervals in my training. The ability to stay calm under pressure, to maintain focus on my goals, and to perform even when faced with adversity has become second nature.

Stubbornness, a quality I've possessed since my training days, serves me well. It's the drive to hustle, to push through the challenges, and to trust myself. I also remind myself to remain open to new possibilities, cultivating curiosity, love, and a thirst for learning. These character strengths build my confidence to face any challenge head-on.

Courage has been my companion throughout life. It fueled my move to New York City at twenty-one, a place where I knew no one. My belief in my protective angels and my hunger for adventure and to be enough guided me. Bravery is intertwined with resilience, helping me navigate physical illnesses and post-traumatic growth.

When the frustrations of personal training became overwhelming, I took a sabbatical. I embarked on a solo bus journey from Puerto Vallarta to Tulum, Mexico, at twenty-three, seeking life lessons. Looking back, I see the courage in my decision to face the unknown, to step out of my comfort zone, and to bet on myself. A gift I gave myself that no one can take.

Understanding and engaging my core has been crucial in my fitness journey. It's not just about preventing injury; it's about fighting gravity as we age. Our bodies are remarkable, and they come equipped with a natural weight belt called the transverse abdominals. Strengthening the core is essential for all forms of exercise, ensuring longevity and sustainability.

Posture plays a significant role in protecting against muscular imbalances, injuries, and aging. Joseph Pilates wisely noted that we're as old as our spine's flexibility. Stiffness and immobility in the spine can affect our entire body's flexibility. To stay agile, we must activate our muscles against gravity.

Flexibility and mobility are often confused. Mobility, the ability to move muscles through a range of motion with control, requires strength. Think of it as the hinge on a door. Mobility exercises focus on joint health and dynamic movements, like leg swings or arm circles. Mobility benefits from dynamic movements, like leg swings, shoulder rotations, or even certain yoga poses that engage multiple joints.

Flexibility is all about your muscles' ability to lengthen. It's like a rubber band stretching—great for static stretches, like touching your toes. Yoga is a fantastic example. For flexibility, think static stretches that hold a position, like touching your toes or a butterfly stretch.

Flexibility for muscles, mobility for joints. Mix both into your routine for a balanced approach to fitness. Remember, it's not just about touching your toes; it's about moving well and staying healthy!

It's about more than just being flexible; it's about master-ing coordination and body awareness. Dynamic stretching is the key, and it's an integral part of maintaining both flexibility and mobility.

During challenging moments, I've learned to speak to myself lovingly and encouragingly. It's a skill honed during strenuous workouts, when I've had to coax myself to start, to focus on each footfall, to engage my core, and to breathe mindfully. Fitness has taught me that it's not about the workout itself; it's about overcoming the struggles it presents, to stay centered no matter what externally is occurring. This cultivated strength has spilled over into my life, helping me find calm and balance amid chaos. It's a moving meditation, a path to inner peace, creating an inner sanctuary and a way to reconnect with my central nervous system.

In life's trying times, remember to be kind to yourself. You have within you the resilience, courage, and strength to overcome any challenge. Use your core, both physical and mental, to stand tall and face the world with confidence. Embrace fitness not just for aesthetics, but for the profound sense of well-being it offers. It might just change your life, as it did mine.

Chapter Six

<hr>

The Magic of Thunder Thighs

"The more grateful I am, the more beauty I see."

~ Mary Davis

In my journey to fitness, there's a significant chapter that revolves around the heat and hills of Hong Kong, where my lifelong love affair with movement began. The sweltering sun bore down on us during afternoon practices, back in the days when sports drinks weren't the norm, and our refreshment was nature's electrolyte-rich gifts—watermelons and oranges. These early memories of using my body, learning discipline, running stairs in the hills with my dog, and building resilience in the relentless heat have shaped the athlete and person I am today.

Hong Kong's tropical climate, with its oppressive humidity, can be daunting to the uninitiated. It's a place where moisture collects on walls like tears, and apartments come equipped with "hot cupboards" to prevent clothes and linens from spoiling. My home was perched on the eleventh floor of an apartment building nestled amidst the island's hills. This setting introduced me to the art of climbing countless stairs and enduring training sessions under the relentless sun. The heat was a constant companion, like an old friend you don't think much about. It never stopped us; it was just part of life, much like the occasional typhoon that would descend upon us, demanding patience, and resilience.

Growing up amidst these weather extremes taught me to thrive in the face of adversity. Heat, typhoons, or any other challenge that came my way was an opportunity for growth. It instilled in me a mentality of embracing discomfort, with the knowledge that storms are fleeting, and the sun will once more grace the sky. It also granted me profound insight into the art of reconstruction after the devastation. It was the foundation for my unshakeable belief in finding solutions rather than dwelling on problems, a trait I later discovered many Floridians shared, a testament to the resilience taught by weather.

My fitness journey began early, involving explosive plyometric training that gave birth to what I affectionately call my "Godzilla thighs." But it wasn't until adolescence that I became conscious of my body's changes and began wrestling with self-doubt. I'd look down at my legs and see quad-zilla muscles and skinny calves, feeling out of place. My perception of my body started to stray from reality, and it marked the beginning of a journey toward self-rejection and comparison with others.

Entering middle school, the quest for acceptance intensi-fied. Middle school, that crucible of teenage angst, where girls were often unkind and boys mystifying. Desperate to belong, I tried to forge friendships with boys but faced ridicule when I refused a kiss, earning the nickname "thunder thighs." This label etched itself into my identity, reinforcing my feelings of inadequacy.

This chapter of my life taught me that our bodies are power-ful allies, and we must be grateful for them. My dad, the wise voice in my life, showed me the path to self-love. He shifted my perspective by reminding me of the privilege of having strong legs, likening them to thunder—nature's warning, a powerful force that brings the heat. This simple mindset shift transformed my self-loathing into appreciation. Every night before bed, my dad and I would kneel, and I'd thank God for my strength and speed, grateful for the gift of my thunder thighs.

Gratitude became a cornerstone of my life, intertwining with my fitness journey. It's a practice that shifts our focus from what we lack to what we have, from self-loathing to self-love. It's the antidote to negative emotions, a way to cultivate resilience, and a means to see beauty even in the most challenging circumstances. I've carried this practice forward into my role as a parent, instilling the habit of "Gratefuls" in my children, and helping them understand the power of seeing the positives in life.

In the heart of New York City, I was young and full of naivetéé when I found myself entangled with a man who resembled a real-life Han Solo. Tall, tanned, and undeniably trendy, I couldn't help but be captivated by his striking appearance. Little did I know that this encounter would serve as a profound lesson, a stark reminder that sometimes we unknowingly adopt stories as our own, without ever questioning their authenticity.

Seated in a chic New York bar, surrounded by a sea of tall, svelte Russian models, our date unfolded. It was there that he uttered those words that would linger in my mind: "Wow! You have big legs."

At that moment, a surge of conflicting emotions coursed through me. A part of me yearned to unleash a torrent of sharp retorts, to school him on the importance of not skipping leg day. But instead, I shrank back, internalizing his words. Later, we found ourselves in his apartment, and I couldn't help but crave his validation, longing for him to see the beauty in me that I couldn't yet see in myself.

This was the very reason I had ventured into the superficial world with this "chicken leg," dude but deep down, I still felt ugly, unworthy, and trapped in the never-ending cycle of comparing myself to the ethereal blonde, waif-like Russian models that surrounded us. Despite my daily prayers of gratitude, a part of my psyche remained ensnared.

As we shared a passionate moment on the couch, I glanced down and noticed that my legs were more substantial than his. In that instant, an unexpected surge of empowerment coursed through me. I knew I couldn't compromise my sense of self and the desires of my heart any longer in the presence of someone who failed to truly understand me.

With newfound resolve, I rose to my feet and declared that I needed someone with thighs even mightier than my own. I yearned for a connection that would ignite both my physical and emotional being, a connection that would hold me close with an intensity that left no room for doubt. I was in pursuit of passion and soulful connection.

Much to my surprise, I never crossed paths with him again. I recall my stoic English mother's voice echoing in my ear, reminding me that what one seeks in a partner at twenty is vastly different from what one seeks at thirty, and evolves once more at forty. The ultimate goal is to find someone who possesses it all and grows alongside you.

And so, from that day forward, I developed a newfound appreciation for training my legs. It became a symbol of my strength and a reminder that true beauty and connection emanate from within.

MUSCLE: YOUR BODY'S FIRE FOR TRANSFORMATION

In the intricate dance of health and fitness, muscle takes center stage, a vibrant performer with multifaceted roles that dictate your body's vitality. Behold its magnificence, for muscle is the beacon that illuminates the path to wellness.

At its core, muscle fuels the metabolic furnace of your being—your Basal Metabolic Rate (BMR). It's the body's voracious calorie consumer, demanding sustenance like no other. A symbiotic relationship emerges the more muscle you nurture, the more calories it demands, harmonizing body fat percentages into a symphony of health.

But muscle's significance transcends the realm of caloric consumption. It weaves a tale of endurance, a tale of hours-long calorie-burning even after the curtains fall on your workout. While the treadmill runner's rhythm dissipates, the muscle-bound continue their fiery performance, crafting a physique that defies the ordinary.

And do not be fooled, for muscle's role isn't confined to aesthetics alone; it safeguards the sanctuary of your bones and organs. In moments of imbalance, falls, and unforeseen adversities, your muscular fortress stands sentinel. It wards off the blows that would otherwise shatter bone and flesh, preserving your vitality in the face of life's capricious nature.

My journey into the world of muscle was seeded in competitive sports, yet I perpetually undermined my own efforts. Olympian dreams remained tantalizingly out of reach, and self-doubt shadowed every stride. Amidst the relentless chase for elusive goals, a quiet voice beckoned me forward, whispering that I was destined for greatness.

Angelic whispers and a steadfast belief in a divine plan guided me, urging me to overcome my self-inflicted obstacles. I needed to learn to train my mind with the same fervor as my body. Thus, I forged a potent elixir of faith, gratitude, and sweat to quell doubt, fear, and negativity.

Gratitude became my steadfast ally, an antidote to the venom of negative emotions. In moments of darkness, it emerged as my guiding light. I channeled the endorphins of high-intensity interval training (HIIT) into a symphony of gratitude for my body's resilience and strength.

Gratitude, a powerful character strength, became the keystone of my mindset. It allowed me to see the vibrant collage of life, transcending the transient woes that tried to confine me. By focusing on the positive, I gained perspective and the ability to rise above challenges.

My daily ritual of gratitude unfurled with the dawn, a harmonious duet with my morning alarm. Before my eyes fluttered open, I serenaded the universe with three notes of thanks. Profound gratitude for another day to embrace my destined path, one more day to serve, and an opportunity to touch lives mired in stories of unworthiness.

In the grand performance of life, muscle is our unerring guide, a burning torch that leads the way to transformation. With faith and gratitude as our faithful companions, we dance to the rhythm of renewal, forging a future defined by strength and vitality.

Throughout my journey, I've met inspiring individuals like a deaf woman I trained. Despite her loss, she radiated strength, courage, and gratitude, teaching me that life's challenges can be transcended through resilience, the desire to create the life you want, and a grateful heart.

As I transitioned into my career as a personal trainer in New York City, I learned the importance of incorporating resistance training into fitness routines. It dispelled the myth that women would bulk up uncontrollably. Building muscle plays a vital role in health and fitness. It elevates your Basal Metabolic Rate(BMR), helping burn more calories, even at rest. It transforms your body into a calorie-burning furnace, thanks to the energy required for muscle repair after resistance workouts.

Muscle-building isn't just about aesthetics; it's about becoming a strong, resilient body capable of handling life's challenges. It provides a protective shield for your bones and organs, a barrier against injuries, aging, and accidents.

My fitness journey is more than just workouts; it's a spiritual practice. It's about summoning the strength to overcome disappointments, embracing challenges, and trusting in a higher plan. In moments of doubt and negativity, I turn to gratitude, shifting my perspective, and rekindling the fire within my heart. It's a reminder that life is a gift, and every day is an opportunity to become the person I choose.

Remember, it's not about dwelling on your body's imperfections but celebrating its strength, capabilities, and growth. Embrace gratitude and change the conversation with yourself from self-loathing to empowerment. Recognize that your body, including your 'thunder thighs,' is a magical, powerful gift from the universe, ready to carry you toward your dreams.

Chapter Seven

Unleashing My Power: Embracing Strength with Boldness

"If you got junk in the trunk, c'mon get low everybody."

~ J-Lo

I was in the bustling heart of NYC, juggling multiple jobs and hustling to make ends meet. Amidst the hustle, a shining moment arrived when I was cast in the coolest off-off Broadway show as a narrator for a captivating Japanese choreographed fight play. I had to be on stage throughout, weaving the story with my words. Our costumes were tight-fitting white attire. Landing this role felt like a monumental achievement, a testament to my talent and hard work.

The anticipation leading up to the first opening night was electric. I couldn't wait to read the reviews, eager to see how they'd praise my performance. But when I finally read them, disappointment washed over me. "The narrator sure does have junk in the trunk," one review quipped. I felt a burning heat rise in my cheeks and a sinking sensation in my stomach. Was that all they saw? My performance had been reduced to a comment about my glutes. It felt like a personal attack, a judgment of my body rather than my talent.

Growing up in Hong Kong, surrounded by peers with slender Asian frames and the era of Kate Moss as the epitome of beauty, I felt hopelessly out of place, a theme for my life. My Portuguese heritage had gifted me with a generous derriere, a trait I'd inherited from my grandmother. She had a full, curvaceous figure well into her 90s, a testament to our genetics.

I struggled to accept my own body, particularly my butt. Embarrassment and shame cloaked my feelings about it. Back then, society had yet to embrace diverse body shapes, especially prominent curves like mine. Unwanted attention, sexual objectification, insensitive comments, and jokes became a part of my daily life. My butt had become my nemesis, a source of shame.

Living in Hong Kong during the annual Rugby Sevens event, I found myself working as a beer girl one year. Our uniforms consisted of short skirts and cute outfits as we sold beer in the stands. During one of my shifts, I overheard someone in the crowd shouting, "Look, there's a cat in her skirt, and it's trying to get out!" Laughter erupted around, fueled by this cruel jest. I was mortified, unable to respond with a clever comeback. The shame clung to me.

In another instance, during a cross-country run, I heard boys behind me making derogatory comments about how my butt seemed to devour my shorts. (yeah, I was in front beating them!) These experiences reinforced the negative narrative I had about my own body.

Having spent over twenty-five years working with women, it pains me to witness how they often speak harshly about their bodies. Our brains tend to fixate on a single negative event, trapping us in an endless cycle of self-doubt and criticism. I've explored various therapeutic approaches, including Acceptance and Commitment Therapy (ACT), which taught me a valuable tool:

THE C-C-C METHOD - CONNECT, CARE, CREATE.
CONNECT

Is about tuning into the sensations in our bodies and acknowledging the emotions they stir. It interrupts the cycle of negative thoughts by offering a new focus for the mind. It aids us to accept that sitting with uncomfortable feelings and not avoid them so they catch up with us later.

CARE

Helps us practice self-compassion and gain perspective on our situation, offering a chance for self-love and personal growth.

CREATE

Empowers us to shift our perspective and choose a more positive emotional response.

By harnessing our character strengths to address these negative emotions, we create new positive experiences and memories. This process, much like a workout, strengthens our ability to embody these strengths, eventually becoming second nature.

J-Lo revolutionized the beauty and fitness industry by proudly embracing her curves. She permitted women to be themselves, to own their bodies, and to be accepted by society. Her journey changed the narrative, liberating women from the confines of unrealistic beauty standards. She remains an iconic figure, using her platform to empower others and even marketing her own booty cream.

When I briefly lived in the vibrant atmosphere of Miami's South Beach, I taught exercise. It became evident how different

New Yorkers and Miami locals were in their approach to fitness. New Yorkers craved guidance and a mind-body connection, while Miami residents just wanted to immerse themselves in music and movement, seeking an escape from the everyday. I learned about a famous surgeon visiting Miami for discreet butt implants, a stark reminder of society's relentless pursuit of beauty. Witnessing the results of cosmetic procedures gone wrong reinforced my commitment to embracing my natural self.

Though the fitness industry often showcases individuals with surgically enhanced bodies, the reality is that many of them suffer from deep self-loathing. I, too, grappled with these issues. Surrounded by this environment, we chase physical beauty and health while emotionally unraveling. My husband played a pivotal role in my journey to self-acceptance. His unwavering support and love became the foundation upon which I rebuilt my self-image.

EMBRACING THE AGELESS BEAUTY WITHIN

As the pages of life turn, and the mirror reflects the milestones of forty-seven years, I find myself at the crossroads of self-acceptance. Genetics have etched laughter lines upon my face, a testament to a life well-lived. The allure of Botox whispers in the background, promising to erase these lines, but my heart remains unwavering.

In the sanctuary of my husband's love, I discovered the true definition of beauty. His words, a tender symphony, remind me daily that I am breathtaking and stunning in my authenticity. " My love, you are absolutely beautifully breathtaking and stunning. Don't try to improve on perfection." His gaze, an unwavering testament to the perfection he sees within me, gently nudges me away from the precipice of self-doubt.

The beauty industry beckons with its siren call, but I am unyielding in my resolve. The prospect of needles dancing upon my skin sends shivers down my spine. I have witnessed the price many in the fitness industry pay, surrendering to surgeries and unhealthy enhancements that mask the deep well of self-loathing beneath. I too, was once entangled in this pursuit of physical perfection, naively believing it could bring me a sense of self-acceptance.

Surrounded by the paradox of sculpted bodies and fractured self-esteem, I chose a different path. My husband's words became my compass, guiding me to wear my face and body with pride, illuminated by the radiance of self-acceptance. If age is etched upon my features, I wear it as a badge of honor, a testament to a life richly lived.

In the hallowed words of the incomparable Jennifer Lopez:

"I just had very low self-esteem. I really believed a lot of what was said, which was I wasn't any good wasn't a good singer, I wasn't a good actress, I wasn't a good dancer-I wasn't good at anything. I just didn't belong here, why wouldn't I just go away?"

I find solace and kinship. Despite her fame and accolades, she too grappled with the weight of self-doubt. Yet, with unyielding bravery, she defied her inner demons, forging a path illuminated by resilience, unwavering commitment, and inspiring bravery.

My training journey led me to the bustling heart of New York City, where a successful client in the fashion world unraveled a poignant narrative. Despite her achievements and elegance, she carried a burden of self-loathing, lamenting her body and succumbing to the allure of surgical interventions. The surgeon's scalpel danced upon her skin, extracting fat from her derrière to fill laugh lines and crow's feet in her face. My heart ached for her as I witnessed her disconnect from her remarkable body.

In those tender moments, I challenged her to speak to herself with the kindness she would bestow upon her daughter. I implored her to nurture her inner child with compassion, love, and encouragement, transforming the harsh monologues into gentle whispers of self-love.

For our bodies are not mere vessels; they are divine instruments bestowed upon us. As women, we bear the miraculous gift of nurturing life within our very beings. Our bodies harbor wisdom beyond our comprehension, a testament to the intricate dance of biology and nature.

Breath, our constant companion, is a sacred gift, a reminder of the miracle of existence. In the throes of life's complexities, we can always find gratitude for this wondrous body that houses our essence, allowing us to be present in this moment.

My profound love affair with my body blossomed on the precipice of meeting my extraordinary husband. His love was the final stroke on the canvas of my self-acceptance. Together, we understood that salvation does not arrive on the shoulders of another; it is our responsibility to heal ourselves. From the crucible of our journeys, we emerged stronger, choosing to heal rather than destroy one another.

In the intricate fabric of life, our bodies are but one thread, woven into the greater narrative of self-acceptance, resilience, and the unwavering commitment to become the best versions of ourselves.

In relationships, we often project our past traumas onto our partners, mistaking them for the people who hurt us in the past. This behavior leads to a cycle of pain and disappointment, but it can be broken through self-awareness and healing. My husband and I experienced this firsthand, coming from backgrounds marked by trauma. We chose to work on ourselves, individually and together. Recognizing that no one else could heal us, we committed to personal growth and mutual support.

Imago therapy taught us the importance of addressing our inner child's wounds and how they influence our adult relationships. It's easy to view your partner as an adversary, especially when you're both carrying the baggage of past traumas. But when we consciously reparent our inner child and provide the safety we lack, the relationship transforms.

Partnerships aren't about expecting your significant other to heal you; they're about becoming each other's allies. We share our stories and baggage, nurturing each other's inner child. It's a profound gift, a journey of healing and growth that my husband and I embarked on together.

At the age of thirty-nine, I found myself pregnant, considered high-risk due to my age. My husband and I owned a CrossFit gym, and I continued with my usual workouts until I experienced bleeding during a challenging workout. Panic set in, and I reluctantly followed my doctor's advice to take it easy. It was a lesson in listening to my body and a stark reminder of my tendency to override its signals.

The hormonal imbalance I faced during pregnancy led to panic attacks and physical symptoms, further emphasizing the importance of the mind-body connection. I realigned myself with my beliefs, recognizing the need for balance and self-compassion.

Optimal performance, I learned from my years of training, requires an ebb and flow. It's about finding the rhythm between pushing and resting. Healing demands a period of rest, allowing us to process our experiences and emerge stronger. In this challenging time, I leaned into the practice of looking for gifts within adversity.

Recently, I faced a setback when I was 'let go' from a job recording exercise videos for a company. This opportunity had felt like a dream come true, but it quickly turned into a challenging experience. Unclear expectations, mixed messages, and a lack of emotional safety in the work environment made it difficult for me to be authentic in front of the camera. Eventually, I received the news that the level of support I required was unsustainable, and I was not being authentic.

It's not uncommon for people to resist those who trigger them or feel threatened by their presence. While the experience was painful, I chose to focus on the knowing rather than the rejection. I knew deep down that this was an opportunity for growth and self-discovery.

Building a thick skin, as they say, is really about strengthening your sense of self and aligning with your moral compass. It's crucial to understand that the only opinion that truly matters is your own. Writing letters to myself has been a helpful practice during difficult times, allowing me to approach my inner dialogue with compassion and love.

Cultivating self-esteem isn't just a concept or affirmation; it's a daily practice. It involves consistent actions and habits that reinforce your worth. It's a journey of overcoming yourself, one day at a time. We must remember that it's not what happens to us but what we do with our experiences that truly matters.

In the face of rejection, I've learned to focus on the knowing, to embrace challenges as gifts, and to guard my moral compass fiercely. Self-esteem is not built on the opinions of others but on our own actions and choices. Each day, we have the opportunity to make ourselves proud.

Embracing adversity and seeking the gifts within challenges has been a recurring theme in my life. The setbacks I've faced have led to growth, self-discovery, and an unwavering faith that something better awaits. Just as in sports, staying in our own lane, playing our own game, and focusing on our goals are essential for success.

Ultimately, the practice of self-compassion and self-acceptance has allowed me to love my body and embrace my unique journey. I've learned that our bodies are truly remarkable, especially when we get out of their way and let them do their magic. Our breath, the gift of life, is a reminder of the wonderment of our bodies.

I've come to cherish my body, especially as I found love with my amazing husband. He became the beacon of self-acceptance in my life, reinforcing my worth and making me feel seen, celebrated, and loved. It took me thirty-seven years to reach a place of resolution and self-love, a place where I no longer had to fight for love.

My journey to self-love has been filled with valuable lessons and transformation. I've come to appreciate the importance of listening to my body, embracing adversity, and cultivating self-esteem through consistent actions. The challenges I've faced have not defined me but have strengthened my resolve to love and accept myself fully.

In the midst of life's tempestuous seas, I've often found solace in a gentle art, writing letters to myself, a tender breeze, Guiding me through each stormy part.

In these pages, I converse with grace Compassion's ink flows an empathetic stream, I speak from the heart, a sacred space, Where love, like moonlight gleams.

From the wellspring of my higher self, from every facet of my being, I draw, a symphony of words, a healing spell, to mend wounds, and strengthen my core.

With kindness as my quill, and love my guide, I navigate life's labyrinthine turns, each letter is a lifeline, a soothing tide, a testament to the resilience within, it yearns. So, in this practice, I find my way, through trials and tribulations, I rise above, and with love and compassion, I'll ever stay, writing letters to myself, an act of self-love.

Dear L,

I wanted to remind you of something truly profound: the twists and turns in life are not regrets; they are the milestones of your extraordinary journey. Each moment, every choice, has contributed to the incredible person you've become.

Let's celebrate those remarkable muscles of yours—they are a testament to your unwavering dedication and tireless work ethic. Don't ever let anyone's opinions or judgments dim the radiant light that is you. If someone can't appreciate your strength, it's simply their loss. Your muscles tell a story of countless hours spent mastering sports, practicing as a child, and pushing your limits. They are a gift from your resilient, hardworking grandparents, a tangible representation of your family's proud legacy.

Always remember, exercise isn't just about aesthetics; it's a sacred privilege, a way to connect with your body, and a path to mental fortitude. It's not a competition to be the fastest or the strongest, nor is it about proving anything to others. It's about nurturing your health, embracing your journey, and fostering your personal growth.

Your muscles are not something to be hidden or ashamed of; they are a testament to your beauty and strength. Your Asian heritage graces your skin with a unique radiance, adding to your distinct allure. Your body is a living canvas, illustrating the story of your origins, your struggles, and your triumphant victories. Your ancestors would undoubtedly swell with pride at your relentless pursuit of improvement and your unyielding determination to shine. But let's not forget that you are so much more than the sum of your physical achievements—you are a beacon of intelligence, wisdom, and constant evolution. Every mistake and lesson has contributed to the incredible person you are today.

Your journey encompasses more than muscles and accomplishments; it's a testament to living a beautiful life and sharing your unparalleled gifts with the world. Your life is a cherished treasure, so seize it, hold it close, and let your brilliant light shine forth.

Always know that I love you, now and for all eternity.

Your Dearest Best Friend,
Laine

Chapter Eight

Resilience in the Empire State: A Journey Through the New York State of Mind

"Do not pray for an easy life, pray for the strength to endure a difficult one."

~ Bruce Lee

When I was acting in New York City, one thing that was always prevalent was that there is no such thing as an overnight success. It takes many nights, moments that the roles cast sometimes had nothing to do with you but who your cast members were and what look they needed, and lots of things needed to align perfectly in order to book the role of your dreams. I did get cast in Law and Order.

I was the lead actor's girlfriend who got murdered. My whole scene was edited out but not the part of me getting strangled to death being found in the snow in Central Park. I remember being in makeup for two hours to perfect a frozen dead look on my skin and a bruised neck. I had to film the snow scene in Central Park. It was literally freezing, and I was partially clothed. If there was any doubt who the girl boss on this show is I can attest it is

Mariska Hargitay. She felt compassion for me lying in the snow and filming. She told production we had to do this scene fast and get 'this poor girl' out of the snow.

After, she came to me and told me I was great and how did I do that.

(Laying in the cold snow, if you remember, I'm a lizard and could bake in the sun all day. Cold is just not my thing.)

I was in the moment and simply replied, "I don't know, state of mind I guess."

She said, "Well, I guess you need to state of mind yourself into the next David Wolfe show."

I smiled and scurried off. Thereafter, I respected this woman and researched her. I saw she has a foundation for abused women. She swam with dolphins at forty and said her life really didn't start till forty. Some of us are late developers, I know I am. I embraced my past as no time was wasted as every lesson, I had I needed to arrive here, now. Having to go through all the experiences we have to in order to learn and implement and grow. The more my life went on this conversation—with this supreme Boss Lady Mariska Hargitay would pop into my head—the more I realized how very profound this was, to be a person that moves others into action, with no expectation. She probably doesn't even remember this conversation or moment, but for me, it was a profound moment etched in my psyche to remember I get to choose my thoughts and have the power to create my life.

Instead of negatively thinking about your body and having self-loathing conversations about your image in the mirror, choose empowering thoughts that move you into action.

Our MINDSET truly creates our reality. What we deeply believe we attract, the deep stories we have told ourselves. Stories born and confirmed by an experience from when we were young are what we take on as our belief system becomes our reality. This perspective forms our realities and the choices we make based on what we believe we deserve. What we believe we become.

This mindset, this way of thinking, is profound for all aspects of our life. It's required for everyone to help us accomplish our task by not giving in or giving up, or it aids in our failures when we tell ourselves we can't make it. New York is known for its hustlers, the grinders who go out every day and push through all the adversities with an end goal in sight. I call this the New York State of Mind that we need to be in. That mindset of nothing is going to stop me! When negative thoughts begin to creep into our heads, we refocus on our goals, remember our why, and push through the current obstacle in our path.

I believe mental fitness is as important as physical fitness. I believe one way of training your mindset is through exercise. Working out allows us to put ourselves under external pressure. Being in a difficult pose or pushing through reps when your body is burning shines a light, and an opportunity to be and observe your thoughts shines a light on how you speak to yourself during external stress. Working out is like our mental training ground. Working out is an opportunity for awareness to change our inner world. You cannot change anything unless are able to see it first. I believe self-awareness, resilience, and mindfulness are emotional muscles that need cultivating just like physical ones.

I've worked in a gym all day for the last twenty years of my life. The majority of my clients are women. It truly breaks my heart to see some of the most physically, and emotionally, talented, beautiful badass women see themselves through the eyes of critical self-loathing. Focusing on things that ultimately don't matter and no one will remember tomorrow. Truly understanding you have the power to change your mind, and how you choose to speak to yourself and see the world, which ultimately creates your experience and your life.

Mindset work is learning to put value in doing the work to change things about your appearance that displeases you equally as important as doing the work to see the beauty in the things you love about yourself. It's learning to expand, change, and flip your perspective. One cannot achieve and maintain an ideal weight without transforming our self-image. One is useless without the other. Engage your body's own ability to rejuvenate itself by being kind, compassionate, and owning your wins instead of criticizing, judging, and turning to negative talk. Choosing to be grateful, instead of hateful towards yourself or your body. Be kind, speak kindly to yourself instead of critically, teach yourself self-progress over perfection and every day little daily habits add up.

When you have a fixed mindset, you cannot grow and expand and you are waiting for things outside your control to create your happiness seeing your failures as permanent. By seeing this way of thinking you can choose to change your attitude, seeing your setbacks, roadblocks, and self-sabotage as stepping stones and as opportunities for improvement and expansion as opposed to rejection and taking the circumstances personally.

To be willing to see your mindset and then want to transform it and change your mindset also involves risks. To speak your truth even if your voice shakes. To have the courage to see risks as opportunities, and the courage to not quit on yourself and complete challenging tasks, to finish what you started, understanding there truly are no such things as shortcuts when you are cultivating and creating a quality, mindset, your body, and lifestyle.

Cultivating a mindset that helps you grow boosts your happiness as you get to make yourself proud and earning anything that helps you feel satisfaction and cultivates a sense of actually liking yourself.

Allow yourself to choose to shine your light brighter to impact the world and give back instead of staying small, focusing on the external, and keep taking. To be able to own your wins, to be able to make yourself ready to receive even more with juicy pleasure and worthiness. It takes willingness, awareness, practice, repetition, compassion, and consistency to cultivate an attitude that is your constant state. Knowing that you are enough exactly as you are! You are exactly where you need to be, working on what you want. Allow yourself to choose to shine your light brighter to impact the world and give back instead of staying small, focusing on the external, and staying stuck.

You also can cope in life when challenging situations arise. You start to look for the solution, see you have choices, and don't stay stuck in disappointment and victimization. You learn to handle setbacks as opportunities and learn tenacity not to quit and approach problems differently. Which helps you appreciate yourself with new eyes and have a sense of self-esteem. Implementing a growth mindset instead of a fixed mindset and taking every opportunity to jujitsu your thoughts until they become muscle memory and find yourself automatically looking for the solution to a circumstance instead of being paralyzed crying over spilled milk.

VALUE PROCESS OVER RESULTS. (THE DAILY WORK, THE HABIT.)

PRACTICE, PROCESS, PRAISE. (CONSISTENCY)

EMBRACE FAILURE MISTAKES AS PART OF LEARNING (WILLINGNESS, COURAGE, ACTION)

SELF-REFLECT AND LEARN THE LESSONS. (THE GIFT)

Your mindset is so much bigger than having abs, squat cleaning a 175-pound barbell, demonstrating the coolest arm balance, obtaining a hundred thousand followers, or earning a billion dollars.

As if you are still operating from fear of not being good enough, being worthy, and not leading with love for yourself and others, you haven't truly won anything because you are constantly at war with the stories in your head telling you that you are not enough. I won't tell you that the stories of not being enough ever truly go away but with awareness and a growth mindset you know how to turn the volume down on these stories and choose a different path other than leading yourself down the path to Harlem within your head. Working to implement the tools that they become skills and know they are not true, and as you overcome and combat them with such voracity and mastery they slowly digress.

Choosing to act, and behaving in a way that leaves you feeling proud of yourself grows your inner relationship with yourself.

What is important is to create your life and your happiness. For me knowing how I feel about myself and how I choose to exchange with others—what I give, and what I was able to receive, ultimately matters at the end of the day. I do know all people remember is not my bank account or abs or followers but how our exchange was.

"Our deepest fear is not that we are inadequate. Our deepest fear is that we are powerful beyond measure. It is our light, not our darkness that most frightens us.

We ask ourselves, 'Who am I? To be brilliant, gorgeous, talented, fabulous?'

Actually, who are you not to be? You are a child of God.

You're playing small does not serve the world.

There is nothing enlightening about shrinking so that other people won't feel insecure around you. We are all meant to shine, as children do. We were born to make manifest the glory of God that is within us. It's not just in some of us; it's in everyone.

And as we let our own light shine, we unconsciously permit other people to do the same.

As we are liberated from our own fear, our presence automatically liberates others." ~ Marianne Williamson

Chapter Nine

The Serenade of Self-Discovery

"God, grant me the serenity to accept the things I cannot change, courage to change the things I can, and wisdom to know the difference."

- Serenity Prayer

My body has always been my vessel, the instrument through which I composed my life's symphony. It was the canvas upon which I painted my emotions and desires, a tapestry of sensations that connected me to the world and all who inhabited it. Every fiber of my being seemed to resonate with profound truth, etching messages into my skin through the language of goosebumps. These messages whispered whether I was safe or needed to escape the clutches of a situation, a place, or a circumstance. An innate intuition guided me, but often, I hesitated, doubting myself, craving external validation more than the whispers of my own spirit.

Too often, I paid dearly for this hesitation, for not fully trusting myself, for sidelining my intuition. The lessons I learned were often costly, and they repeated until I accepted accountability, untangling the threads of blame from the fabric of my growth. The beauty industry, with its relentless pursuit of an unattainable standard of flawlessness, engraved this notion of inadequacy into my subconscious from a young age.

Throughout these lessons, however, a profound sense of being loved persisted within me, not just by my biological parents but by the universe itself, by the very spirit that bound us all. I couldn't perceive this during the trials, but in the aftermath of healing, I came to recognize that every mistake and every person sent to teach me were divine gifts. These individuals, the bearers of lessons, were my spiritual angels in disguise. I couldn't see it then, but their purpose was to lead me toward growth and illumination, like celestial guides in the intricate dance of my existence.

Yet, entangled in a web of self-doubt, my relationships were chaotic, lacking consciousness. I was drawn to chaos because, deep down, I held the belief that I was not enough.

I found myself in a relationship with a man who embodied every quality a woman, especially myself, could desire. He was the ideal father figure, and he loved me despite my emotional turbulence. We reveled in the joy of everyday life, laughing together, and sharing our dreams. He'd tell me he adored every facet of me, and I, in turn, found comfort in his love. Yet, the very depth of his love for me frightened me to my core. Little did I know then that my nervous system was a battlefield, waging a war between trauma and reason.

A part of me perpetually yearned to end the relationship, convinced that I didn't deserve the love he poured upon me. Deep down, I feared that he would stop loving me if he discovered the real me, the imperfect me. I was profoundly immature and scarred, entangled in daily emotional turmoil, and I inadvertently hurt him, betraying his love and reinforcing my own self-doubt.

They say hurt people hurt people, and I hurt many good souls who saw me for who I was and loved me deeply anyway. I was wounded, desperately trying to prove them wrong. As I've grown and embarked on my healing journey, I've come to realize that I couldn't have acted differently at the time. I genuinely believed I didn't deserve such love, and I'd go to great lengths to confirm my self-imposed verdict. I was a lovable mess, leaving a trail of collateral damage in my wake.

I also harbored the self-awareness that I had much inner work to undertake. I remember this kind-hearted, funny man dropping profound truths on me. One day, he uttered, "You care more about six-pack abs than being treated like a queen." His words struck like lightning, revealing how I had lived on the surface of my existence, fearful of vulnerability and honesty, both with myself and my partners. Thus, I sought happiness in dysfunctional, toxic, and tumultuous relationships.

He also gifted me with another insight. "You exercise every day, but it never changes your body." At that point, I hadn't ventured into weightlifting or become a trainer, but his words resonated deeply within me. I recognized that true change required different actions, and a willingness to step into discomfort. Thus, I began lifting weights, sculpting my body, and delving into the art of body composition transformation. This kind-hearted man, whom I loved but didn't know how to love, left an indelible mark on my soul.

Understanding that love is an action, a daily choice, proved to be an epiphany. This man profoundly influenced the woman I would become, offering me a glimpse of the kind of partner I desired in life and the vision of a conscious, loving relationship. He made me feel beautiful, and I couldn't fathom how he saw me until I rebuilt my own self-esteem.

Tears often flowed in his presence, a testament to his ability to make me feel safe. Unbeknownst to me then, my central nervous system perpetually existed in a state of fight or flight, and his love triggered a physiological response, moving me to tears of profound acceptance. Yet, I couldn't extend this same compassion and love to myself; I didn't feel worthy. No amount of rational thought could override this physiological sensation. I yearned for somatic healing, for a way to bridge the disconnect between my body and spirit.

Since childhood, I had awakened with a nervous tummy, a daily apprehension. This sensation was a language my central nervous system spoke, signaling its unrest. Somatic therapies emerged as the key to deciphering these messages, connecting my mind and body through touch and movement. They trained my nervous system to embrace bodily cues and sensations, replacing fear with familiarity. Somatic therapy addresses muscular tension, digestive issues, sleep disturbances, respiratory challenges, chronic pain, and imbalances. It was a practice that hinged on the belief that our bodies retained every memory and that unresolved trauma lingered in our physical form.

Even now, at forty-seven, I occasionally wake with that familiar nervous sensation in my stomach. When it happens, I practice self-soothing and reiki, granting myself a moment to engage with the fear triggered by a situation. It's about learning to listen to my body, responding with love, kindness, and space, empowering me to face challenges with pride, with the ability to respond rather than succumbing to a trauma-induced reaction.

This journey led me to explore various forms of somatic exercise: Rolfing (structural integration), Juicing, Reiki, Yoga, Breathwork, Dance, Pilates, Acupuncture, Alexander technique, Gyro-tonics, Feldenkrais method, and Laban movement.

I've always held the belief that knowledge is power, and in a world awash with information, we have the choice to remain ignorant or bewildered, or we can simplify and apply what resonates with our individual selves. I share these experiences, hoping they may guide others who grapple with anxiety or other mental health challenges.

My ACT therapist became a beacon of light during a turbulent phase in my life. I questioned everything—myself, my health, my abilities—while emerging from a toxic, gas-lighting relationship that had left me disoriented and lost. My ex-partner's relentless social drug dabbling, functioning alcoholism and verbal abuse and name-calling abusive behavior and choices had upended my sense of self. I was adrift, doubting my very sanity.

I sought my therapist's guidance, asking if I might be bipolar, and requesting tests to determine my mental state. Her response was illuminating. She explained that every person on this planet carries trauma; it's how we cope with it that matters. She also taught me that every person on this planet possesses traits that could be labeled as borderline personality disorder, but the crucial distinction lies in embracing or resisting those traits that decipher our actions and choices. Together, we embarked on a journey to heal my heart and train my mind, address my traumas, and assume responsibility for my choices and experiences, so I could learn from them and thus have the freedom to choose differently. This newfound strength empowered me to fight for myself and the people I loved, vowing never to abandon myself for another soul. The way we digest our thoughts, I realized, is just as vital as how we digest our food.

Chapter Ten

———◦●◦———

Mindful Eating, Body Love, and Personal Growth

"The Body becomes what the foods are. As the spirit becomes what the thoughts are."

~ Ancient Kemetic Proverb

Let's talk food. To start with... EVERYONE is not on the same path, in any way. Therefore, our nutritional needs are going to be different along with our workout needs. Keep that in mind throughout this journey!

Many times, our food can trigger responses in our body, and we ignore the signals and/or refuse to hear them. Eating is an act of self-love and self-respect, and if we could have a spiritual connection to our food—understanding and knowing where it comes from and how it is grown, raised, and produced—allow us to see the privilege of eating and to look at it as such. Eating with gratitude—a mindset of nourishing our bodies and digesting our food with love and gratitude—will make it easier to digest than eating from motivations of mindless distractions, guilt, self-harm, overeating to fill a void, boredom or an inability to sit in the emptiness of that emotion at that moment, greed, over-indulgence, and closet eating. I have seen many of these situations with my clients. We try to add the exercise of eating mindfully and intuitively and listening to your body while achieving a certain body composition.

A question I get asked frequently: "I don't want to lose muscle (or want to build more muscle), what should I do?"

Answer—Nutrition Side: Make sure that when you eat, every "meal" has a source of protein in it! Quick choices would be lean ground beef, chicken, and fish. Those are your basic straight protein sources. There are several other foods from the carb and fats family that have high protein values in them as well (quick example: eggs, nuts—fat with protein—and quinoa—high carb with protein). In a nutshell, focus on healthy veggies for carbs, keep fruit consumption on the lighter side (one to two servings), choose healthy fats (nuts, seeds, avocado, salmon, olive oil, for example), and include a palm-sized protein serving. Save some carbs for after your workout (rice is a good choice here) to replenish the glycogen levels in your body. Add some protein in for muscle repair (oh yeah, we are still working our muscles doing cardio!) Losing "weight," as we like to say, is all about calories in versus calories out. In simpler terms, if you eat fewer calories than you burn, you lose weight. However, it's crucial to understand your own body and its unique needs.

We know that nutrition is vital for all things, be it losing weight, toning, gaining muscle, or even having more energy and a better overall sense of health and wellness. While many diets can help you lose weight, the diet you choose should fit your lifestyle and health demands and have longevity and sustainability as keywords, with your food preferences in mind. Ultimately, it's about choosing a diet that works for your body and your life. At the end of the day, you choose what you put in your mouth.

So, ask yourself: Are you willing to do what is necessary to achieve the results you want?

Answer Workout Side: You need to lift weights and not be scared of it. Let's get one thing straight: It's not as easy to gain muscle as some might think! The number one thing I've heard for the last twenty years is "I don't want to get big muscles!" The number of women I've trained that ended up with "manly" muscles equals zero. Can it be done? Sure. But you have to train hard, eat right, and strive to build muscle like that. It doesn't come easy, not even for men with higher testosterone levels! So, don't worry about something that's never going to happen, and let's work toward attaining those goals!

Focus your workouts around a hypertrophic environment (we'll call this the "muscle-building zone"). We need to move weight that's in the range of six to twelve reps—meaning a weight you can do between six to twelve reps of—work sets, and give rest in between those sets. You have to stress the muscle, allow it to recover, and stress it again. Rest should be between sixty to ninety seconds between sets. Sets are groups of reps (stay with me here). You can work on muscle groups or your whole body.

MUSCLE GROUPS EXAMPLE:

Chest and Triceps

- Dumbbell bench press: 5 sets of 8-10 reps
- Push-ups: 3 sets of up to 12 reps (STRICT form)
- Dumbbell kickbacks: 3 sets of 10 reps on each arm (flex at the end of each rep)
- Banded triceps pushdown: 3 sets of 12-15 reps (elbows stay locked in place)

TOTAL BODY EXAMPLE:

- Dumbbell Bench Press 4 sets of 10 reps
- Back squat 4 sets of 8-10 reps
- Chin-ups 4 sets of up to 8 reps
- Sumo Deadlift: 4 sets of 8-10 reps
- Dumbbell lateral raises: 3 sets of 10 reps
- Dumbbell hammer curl: 3 sets of 8-10 reps
- Banded triceps pushdown: 3 sets of 12 reps
- V-Up: 4 sets of 12-15 reps
- Dumbbell Russian Twist: 2 sets of 20 reps

THE PLUSES AND MINUSES OF EACH:
TOTAL BODY:

This method generally comes with a little more volume in the workout. Three times a week would be enough. It doesn't allow for a lot of total muscle destruction, therefore allowing you to train that muscle again in a shorter timeframe. It generally results in a slightly higher heart rate due to the volume of training, which burns some extra calories during the workout. If you don't have four to five days a week for working out, this allows you to cover it generally in three. Plus, if you miss a day, you don't miss an entire muscle group!

MUSCLE GROUP:

This method requires more discipline in the way you need to work out each day, or you might end up missing an entire muscle group as you only hit muscle groups once per week. When you do hit them, you stress them to the maximum, allowing for maximum rest to recover and repair. This method also allows more time to incorporate different angles of training for individual muscles.

Ultimately, it's all about your goals, your commitment level, and your individual body. Remember, it's not a one-size-fits-all journey, and nobody knows your body better than you do when you have invested the time to learn it and listen to it. Take the time to be open to trying new things and experiment with what works best for you.

To reach your fitness goals, keep it simple and make sure you include squats, deadlifts, unilateral single-limb movements, pushing, pulling, and pressing in your training routine focusing on quality movement patterns is vital, creating a mind-body awareness and mind-muscle connection.

In the vibrant heart of New York City, amidst the pulsating energy of the underground gym scene, I embarked on a journey that would teach me invaluable lessons about self-worth, resilience, and the power of choice. It was a place where the pursuit of perfection knew no bounds, and the pressure to conform to society's ideals extended beyond gender lines.

As I ventured deeper into this world, I encountered individuals who had undergone drastic transformations in their quest for physical perfection. Calf implants, pec implants, and a relentless pursuit of an impossible standard of beauty were the norms here. It was in this chaotic and passionate environment that I stumbled upon a life-altering lesson—a lesson about choosing conscious, healthy relationships over tumultuous and destructive ones.

In the midst of this whirlwind, I found myself drawn to a man whose emotional wounds ran deep. His turbulent past and the traumas he had endured were etched into his soul, leaving him emotionally fractured. Despite the glaring red flags and the warning signs, I convinced myself that I could love him into healing, that I could save him from his demons. I was trapped in a cycle of dysfunction and abuse, seeking external validation and affirmation from someone incapable of giving it, even to himself.

Our relationship was a toxic dance of codependency and abuse. The more I tried to fix him, the more I lost myself. It was a chaotic, destructive spiral, and we were both emotionally immature, projecting our wounds onto each other. It wasn't just about him; it was about me—why I believed I deserved to be treated this way, why I couldn't break free from the cycle.

But the universe had other plans. It intervened, forcing a geographical separation that became the catalyst for my healing journey. I was physically and emotionally drained, covered in hives from the cortisol coursing through my body. I had sacrificed my career, my home, my financial stability, and even my beloved cats and the idea of what I thought my life was going to be. It was a rock bottom that served as the foundation for my transformation.

This relationship had stripped away my survivor mask, exposing my vulnerabilities and insecurities. I felt the pain of abandonment in every fiber of my being, but I refused to succumb to it. I knew I could rise above the darkness, that healing was possible. I sought therapy, surrounded myself with loved ones, and embraced the lessons life had to offer.

Healing wasn't easy. It required me to dig deep into my past, to acknowledge the trauma bonds that had kept me trapped. I had to forgive myself for my decisions, to accept responsibility for my choices. It was about understanding that the blame game would never set me free, and that true transformation began with self-love and self-acceptance.

I embarked on a journey of self-discovery, anchored by affirmations and self-love practices. I learned to hold myself accountable for my actions and reactions and to envision the woman I wanted to become. It was a conscious effort to nurture a loving relationship with myself, to rewrite my story, and to let go of the past.

At forty-six, I faced a significant milestone—a breast explant surgery. It was a symbolic act of self-love and acceptance, a farewell to the physical alterations I had once believed would bring me happiness. The surgeon revealed that my body had formed a protective capsule around a ruptured implant, a testament to the resilience and wisdom of the human body. As I lay on the cusp of surgery, the anesthesiologist's words resonated deeply, "It's funny how, as we age, our desires change, and it's not about priorities, but wisdom. What we crave when we're young isn't what we cherish as we grow older. To discern those desires with insight is the true essence of wisdom."

From this experience, I've learned not to forsake myself for an unattainable standard of beauty achieved through chemicals and foreign objects. Instead, I've come to value the beauty found in nurturing qualities, characteristics, and depth within, sharing my authentic self with the world. Recognizing my intrinsic worth and persisting through adversity, that, to me, is genuine beauty.

In embracing my scars, both physical and emotional, I have found my strength. My journey through chaos and self-discovery has led me to a place of self-love, where I proudly declare, "I love myself, all of me—from my past choices to the woman I am becoming."

It took years for me to recognize the importance of listening to my inner spirit, having the confidence to act on it, and trusting myself. I learned that self-love and acceptance were not achieved through external changes but through inner growth and self-awareness.

One of the most significant lessons I learned during this journey was the power of mindfulness. It was essential to be present in the moment, to appreciate my body, and to eat mindfully, not as a way to numb emotions or seek comfort but as a way to nourish and love myself. I realized that mindful eating was a form of self-care and self-compassion.

Practicing self-love and personal growth required embracing vulnerability and authenticity. It meant being open to my imperfections and accepting myself wholly, flaws and all. It meant acknowledging that growth was a continuous process and that self-love was not a destination but a lifelong journey.

I also found strength in community and support. Connecting with others who shared similar struggles and goals was incredibly empowering. It reminded me that I was not alone in my journey, and there was strength in unity and shared experiences.

My journey to self-love, body acceptance, and personal growth was filled with valuable lessons. It taught me the importance of mindful eating, the significance of embracing my true self, and the power of vulnerability and authenticity. It was a journey of self-discovery and self-compassion, and it continues to be a path I walk with gratitude and love for myself.

Chapter Eleven

---•◆•---

Limitless Valor: No Expiry in Sight

"Embrace every moment of your life, for time never takes a break, and dreams know no expiry date."

~ Satyabati Swain

Our perception of what our bodies should be is often clouded by misconceptions, causing us to seek control over the outcome instead of appreciating the rewards of our hard work and genetic potential. My body has a natural predisposition to build muscle quickly. My legs, sculpted from years of college field hockey and sprinting across the Astro-turf field, always made me self-conscious about having larger legs than most women (and even some men) around me. Whenever I noticed my traps or biceps gaining size, the fear of "I'm getting too bulky" would creep in, leading me to reduce the intensity of my weight training to maintain control over my physique's narrative and outcome.

The true key to success is self-awareness: knowing your body, experimenting to find what works best for your unique body chemistry, and embracing the journey.

Understanding the pivotal role of nutrition in achieving all your goals, whether it's losing weight, toning up, gaining muscle, or simply feeling healthier, is one thing. Putting this knowledge into practice is another. While pizza, cake, and wine might pro-vide instant gratification, they won't sustain you for optimal daily performance, recovery, and emotional well-being. You might ask, "How do I determine how much to eat?" We're about to dive deep into this, so take a deep breath and follow along until you've explored the depths.

Every person has a Basal Metabolic Rate (BMR), which repre-sents the number of calories your body burns each day by merely existing. Muscles and organs require energy and nutrients to function, and this energy depends on your muscle mass and daily activity levels (excluding exercise for now). Your BMR serves as the baseline for your daily calorie consumption: eat at this level, and your weight remains constant; consume less, and you lose weight; consume more, and you gain weight. Additionally, burn-ing extra calories through exercise can help with weight loss.

MUSCLE is what determines your Metabolic Rate (how many calories your body burns just being you). The less muscle, the fewer calories (energy) your body needs. Now we are spin-ning wheels... On top of that, not only are you making it harder to lose body fat, but you're also creating your body's metabolism to run inefficiently and ineffectively. Your body is smarter than you. It's GOING to stay alive! The next time you consume more calories than your body needs at that moment, it's going to store the remainder of those calories instead of excreting them. And you know how it stores it, don't you? As FAT!

I've come to love the feeling of pushing my limits, discov-ering my body's endurance, and witnessing its capabilities. My love shifted from being result-oriented to embracing the pro-cess itself—the confidence that consistent effort, guided by my genetic potential, would yield results. I learned that I had to relin-quish control over every outcome, stop trying to fit my body into an unrealistic mold through dieting or training and embrace my body's natural form. I have hips, a waist, and thighs; I was never meant to be a Kate Moss. I've seen many women trying to force a square peg into a round hole, not only regarding their bodies but also in their relationships and expectations of how things should be. Instead of accepting reality, they persist in unhealthy eating and unsustainable workout routines, marked by unrealistic goals and high price tags. I realized that health and fitness have no expiration date. By training in a way that promotes longevity, sustainability, and joy, based on my genetic potential, my body evolved into what it was meant to be. It's akin to being gifted with talent and working diligently to maximize it.

Many stories exist of people involved in car accidents, leaving the hospital after X-rays, only to discover later that they had a broken neck. If not for their well-developed traps from weight training, they might have been paralyzed for life. Muscle is not the enemy; it contributes to a healthy body, a robust metabolic system, and something to be thankful for as we age.

As I let go of my fear of having too much muscle, I started taking pride in my body's strength and appreciated how resilient and powerful I felt. My loving and supportive husband reassured me of my attractiveness, emphasizing how hot he found me, with my soft brown skin, womanly curves, and athletic tone. He made me feel safe on a deep, cellular level, allowing me to honor and cherish my body's strength, beauty, and resilience, enabling me to be truly vulnerable in our relationship. I found a newfound freedom in every aspect of my life, trusting the universe at a profound level. I realized that if I consistently brought my best self to each day, the results would follow—the form of results, not forced into my preconceived idea of what they should be. This liberation meant no longer trying to squeeze into a size six shoe when I'm a size seven in every aspect of life. I learned to accept what is, shedding unnecessary suffering and excess.

If you're still uncertain about building muscle, I understand. But there's a significant difference, both in nutrition and training, between developing a strong, muscular physique and training for a bodybuilding competition.

Another common question is, "I want to look like I work out but not like a bodybuilder. How do I achieve that?"

The quickest way to achieve a fit appearance is by building muscle. It not only enhances aesthetics but also strength. There's a substantial contrast between someone with a strong, muscular physique at the pool and the same person training for a bodybuilding competition. They don't look the same, despite both having muscular builds. Looking like a bodybuilder takes immense discipline in training, nutrition, and hard work, especially for women. It doesn't happen accidentally through weight training; it requires dedication, sacrifice, and consistency. So, there's no need to worry about that. Focus on eating enough to support muscle growth to attain a toned, athletic appearance.

To understand muscle building better, let's have a quick crash course. Muscles need specific "supplies" to grow, just like building a house. Timing is crucial. One often underestimated factor in aesthetics is glycogen replenishment, which can be achieved by consuming simple carbohydrates post-workout (within thirty minutes). This increases blood sugar levels, prompting the release of insulin, an anabolic hormone that aids muscle protein synthesis.

Additionally, you require the building blocks for muscle growth—protein. Protein is the essential ingredient for muscle building. Without enough protein, you could do everything else correctly and still achieve nothing. Aim to consume at least 1 gram of protein per pound of body weight.

When people ask how I got my arms, glutes, or physique, I often remind them that it's the result of over three decades of consistent effort. It wasn't my initial goal when I started. I showed up because it became part of me—a daily ritual that supported my mental health, served as my moving meditation, and allowed me to choose myself every day. It was my escape from codependency, a path to self-discovery, and a testament to my commitment to personal growth.

The journey isn't about achieving a predefined outcome—it's about embracing the process and allowing your body to become its best self. In the end, there's no expiration date on your health and fitness. So, show up, offer your best self daily, and watch the results unfold in their unique and beautiful form.

Chapter Twelve

Unveiling Destiny: Unlocking the Golden Gate

"In the grand theater of life, it's not the hand you're dealt that defines you; it's how you choose to play it."

- Randy Pausch

Consistency is the golden key that unlocks the gates to your health and well-being. It's in the daily choices, the unwavering commitment, and the persistent actions that we find the path to the life we envision.

Within each of us, there's a battle. It's not a simple question; it's a profound one: "Do you truly desire to become the healthier, leaner version of yourself?" This answer only you can provide. But let me assure you, as this commitment transforms into a habit, you'll witness the remarkable difference in how you feel, the way your clothes fit, and the confidence that grows within you.

In the beginning, the battle rages within. But don't fear this inner turmoil; instead, embrace it. Discover what ignites your passion and fuels your determination to win each skirmish. Find your resounding *Why*—the reason that keeps you committed, despite the challenges. Remember, commitment isn't about wanting to reach your goals; it's about how fiercely you want them.

Starting out, it's easy to declare, "I'm going to work out and shed those extra pounds! I'll regain my youthful form!" In that moment, you're inspired, motivated, and filled with intent. But then comes tomorrow, the reality check. The alarm rings, and that same enthusiasm has vanished. An inner voice whispers, "Just five more minutes in bed," or "You can't do this; you know you won't last." It's a pivotal moment—the crossroads between commitment and comfort.

Your date with your healthier self—is it more important than those extra minutes of sleep? Another glass of wine? Late-night snacks? Planning your meals and workouts while everyone else indulges in pizza and pasta—is that your priority? Do you truly want to embrace the leaner, healthier you more than remaining as you are?

Remember the vision of yourself, the feeling of accomplishment, and the pride that surged when you visualized your goal. Each morning, you must recapture that sensation, for this journey won't be easy. It's a promise—there will be days you'll resist exercise, moments when fatigue seems insurmountable, and cravings that beckon you towards indulgence. Those are the days when you must silence the inner naysayers and summon your inner champion.

Exercise is often the easier part; it's the eating that presents the real challenge. Choosing the right foods, controlling portion sizes, and resisting temptations can be a Herculean task. Remember, if your goal is 70% nutrition, then it's precisely that—not 60%, not 80%, but 70%. You can hit the gym, give it your all, and still fail if you neglect your diet. Being aware, accountable, and making a plan is much better than being led blindly by impulse, emotion, or reacting to your hunger when it strikes. So, when you see me or anyone who has had the same success as I have, it has come down to creating balance, consistency, and accountability, not just in the exercise realm.

Failure to plan your nutrition is a plan to fail. It helps to get clear with how much you are actually consuming by implementing a system of recording for a week to be able to take measurements of what you are actually consuming whether it's with precise numbers or a more intuitive approach to stay aware. Consistency reigns supreme in your journey to progress. Tracking your food holds you accountable, preventing mindless consumption. It doesn't have to be rigid, but it does require awareness of what you're putting into your body.

You aren't perfect, and that's okay. What matters is that you track your food, honestly and consistently. Consistency is the cornerstone of progress. There are no shortcuts to success; it's a path that demands effort and commitment.

If you're serious about making your goals, then you need to be serious about what you are consuming (how much and learning to trust your intuition). Eating too much we put weight on; eating too little you don't give yourself enough gas (food). Your body isn't going to shut down on the side of the road (it will, just not immediately), it's going to find gas! And it needs gas NOW, not later, because you keep moving, walking around, getting excited while talking, etc., and the fastest thing your body can do to create gas is burn muscle tissue!

The journey towards a healthier you is unique, and there are various eating styles to explore. You need to find the one that suits your lifestyle and sets you up for success. Your food choices shape your results, so keep it simple. From intuitive eating to macro counting, each approach has its merits. The key is discovering what works best for your body and lifestyle.

Intuitive eating is akin to trusting your gut. Listen to your body's hunger and fullness cues, and make balanced meal choices. Rid yourself of the notion that there's a one-size-fits-all solution. Experiment, learn, and adapt to what your body responds to best.

Understanding macronutrients—proteins, carbohydrates, and fats—is crucial.

Proteins repair and build tissue, carbohydrates fuel your brain and body, and fats are essential for nutrient absorption. It's not about eliminating them; it's about finding the right balance.

I have done macros, and they produce great results. But I don't find them feasible for my lifestyle with kids and their schedules, measuring, cooking, training, and being on my phone measuring and recording. I prefer an intuitive eating style; this is where I listen to my body, use hand measurements, and strive towards living a balanced life. (This took time and experimenting with different methods of what worked for me and the results I was looking for.) Anything new we start is a learning curve, especially when you're learning about your own body and what works for you and trusting yourself. No one knows your body better than you when you listen to it.

Remember, the health and fitness industry is a multi-billion-dollar industry that counts on you being confused to make moolah off you. It is rare for any multi-billion-dollar industry to teach you to be empowered. They don't teach you to be self-reliant, self-motivated, to be intuitive, and strive for balance as there is no sell in that. We all know what to do, and we all really know how to do it. You can accomplish ANYTHING you want if you decide that's what you WANT to do!

If you want it, be willing to do all the things it takes to accomplish it (might mean changing your mindset on what you are eating. Might mean being honest with what you are eating. Might mean asking for help, hiring a coach, or signing up for meal delivery plans—it looks different for everyone—it is simple, but if we make it complicated, it helps with the excuses to continue to stay the same), not just the things you like to do.

Make it fun! Make it a date. It should be fun! Don't make it just about losing weight or being on a diet. Make it about striving for a healthier lifestyle. The weight loss or getting stronger is just the outcome of getting healthier and creating lifelong sustainable habits that you can continue for the rest of your life. Remember what got you in the shape you were before. Lifestyle, habits, and choices. It is OK to enjoy life and have food that is considered off the 'healthy' scale, but you just have to be aware of the consequences of your choices and plan your day around them.

Each of us is unique, and what works for one may not work for another. Experiment with different approaches, and don't be afraid to tailor your nutrition to your individual needs. Your body is your responsibility; get to know it intimately.

In the realm of health and fitness, simplicity often trumps complexity. Don't let the profit-driven industry confuse you; you have the power to understand your body. You can achieve anything if you decide that's what you truly want. Be willing to make the necessary changes, seek help when needed, and trust the process. Balance is the key to sustainability, longevity, and consistency. Balance may not be easy, but it's a worthy pursuit.

For lasting change, you must become a different person. Visualize the qualities you need to manifest your desires. Your thoughts are the language of your brain, and your feelings are the language of your body. Take control of your day, starting with your first waking moments. Rise with intention, not obligation. Break free from the body's desires and let your mind and your chosen habits guide you.

Gratitude is a potent tool in this journey. Reflect on what you're grateful for, and send out gratitude to the world. The power of the mind is incredible—it can heal, transform, and manifest. The placebo effect proves that we can heal ourselves through the power of thought and emotion. Embrace the science behind it and cultivate a mindset of wellness.

Choose to be greater than your environment. Define yourself by your vision, not your circumstances. Review your choices daily and take actions aligned with your vision. The power lies in being defined by the future you aspire to, not the past that holds you back.

Create conscious self-creations which are affirmations in the present that reinforce the woman you want to become. This is bridging the gap for your present self to your future self. Write them, see them, read them, say them, hear them, believe them, feel them, live them. You are not defined by your thoughts, fears, failures, or limitations; you are defined by your actions and choices.

Challenges are not about losing a set amount of weight in a short time. They should focus on cultivating daily habits that lead to lasting transformation. Small daily choices accumulate into profound results.

What do I eat? There are various eating styles, but the key is to find what suits your lifestyle. Intuitive eating lets you trust your body's signals of hunger and fullness. Pay attention to these cues, eat balanced meals, and reject the diet mentality.

Understanding macros—proteins, carbohydrates, and fats— is vital. Each macronutrient serves a purpose, and finding the right balance for your body is essential. Experiment, adapt, and learn what works best for you.

In your unique journey to health, simplicity reigns supreme. The health and fitness industry thrives on confusion, but you possess the wisdom to discern what's right for you. Take the time to understand your body, listen to its needs, and simplify your path to lasting health and well-being. You hold the power to shape your destiny—one choice, one action, at a time.

There are no shortcuts on the path to success!

Chapter Thirteen

The Power of Consistency: Unleash Your Inner Warrior

"Consistency is the mother of mastery."

~ Robin Sharma

Consistency is your secret weapon, your North Star in the realm of health and fitness. It's not about perfection but about the unwavering commitment to those small, sustainable choices that propel you toward your goals.

Consistency is the most powerful tool in your arsenal when it comes to making lasting changes to your body and health. Consistency is about making small, sustainable choices that create your daily habits. When you're consistent, you build habits. These habits become second nature, and you no longer have to think about them. Eating healthy and exercising regularly become as automatic as brushing your teeth or tying your shoes.

In the end, your fitness journey is not just about the destination; it's about the journey itself. It's about the person you become along the way, the lessons you learn, and the growth you experience.

Picture this: by practicing you etch healthy habits into your daily routine so seamlessly that they're as automatic as tying your shoelaces. Nourishing your body and engaging in regular exercise become as integral to your day as breathing itself.

Consistency is what separates the people who achieve their goals from those who don't. It's easy to get motivated and excited about a new diet or exercise program, but that initial burst of motivation will only take you so far. It's the daily grind, the commitment to showing up even when you don't feel like it, that ultimately leads to success.

Here's the undeniable truth: consistency separates the dreamers from the achievers. Sure, that initial burst of motivation can ignite a fire within you, but it's the everyday hustle, the unyielding dedication even when motivation wanes, that will define your success.

As you embark on this transformative journey, here are some sage tips to guide you:

SET REALISTIC GOALS

Don't set yourself up for failure by setting goals that are too ambitious. Start with small, achievable goals and gradually work your way up. Begin with attainable objectives, and gradually elevate the bar. Rome wasn't built in a day, and neither are strong, healthy bodies.

CREATE A SCHEDULE

Plan your workouts and meals and stick to a schedule. Treat your workouts with importance like appointments that can't be missed. Most importantly, be kind to yourself. Don't compare your progress to others, and don't be too hard on yourself when things don't go as planned. You are a work in progress, and that's okay. What matters is that you keep moving forward, one step at a time, toward a healthier and happier you.

FIND ACCOUNTABILITY

Whether it's a workout buddy, a coach, or a support group, having someone to hold you accountable can make a big difference.

TRACK YOUR PROGRESS

Keep a record of your workouts and meals. This can help you see how far you've come and stay motivated. Document your journey. Reflecting on how far you've come is both empowering and motivating.

FOCUS ON THE PROCESS

Instead of obsessing over the end result, focus on the daily actions that will get you there. Celebrate small victories along the way. Resist the temptation to dwell solely on the endgame. Instead, savor the daily actions that will usher you toward your goal. Celebrate each small victory as a stepping stone.

STAY FLEXIBLE

Life happens, and there will be days when you can't stick to your plan perfectly. That's okay. The key is to get back on track as soon as possible. Life is unpredictable, and curveballs are inevitable.

On days when your plan goes awry, adapt, and get back on track as soon as possible.

LEARN FROM SETBACKS

Embrace the challenges and setbacks as opportunities for growth. Every time you face an obstacle and overcome it, you become stronger and more resilient. Don't be afraid to step out of your comfort zone and try new things. You might discover a passion for a type of exercise or a healthy recipe that you never knew existed. When you stumble, view it as a lesson rather than a failure. Every setback is an opportunity for growth.

STAY PATIENT

Consistency takes time to pay off. Be patient and trust the process. Learn to enjoy the process of taking care of your body. It's not a punishment; it's a gift you give yourself. Celebrate your successes, no matter how small they may seem. Be proud of every workout you complete, every healthy meal you eat, and every positive choice you make.

Remember, the path to a healthier, fitter you is a lifelong endeavor, a marathon, not a 30-day challenge or sprint. Trust the process, and don't be disheartened by setbacks.

EVERY STEP FORWARD IS PROGRESS.

Keep in mind, your journey is a testament to your strength and resilience. It's not just about reaching your destination; it's about evolving into the best version of yourself.

Embrace the power of consistency, for it will be your unwavering ally in this extraordinary expedition. Stay the course, and soon, you'll stand triumphantly at the peak of your potential, looking back at the incredible journey you undertook.

Remember, you have the power to transform your body and your life. It all starts with a decision, a commitment, and the willingness to take action. So, are you ready to embark on your own fitness journey? The road may be long, but the destination is worth every step. Start today, and never look back.

YOUR HEALTH AND FITNESS SELF LOVE JOURNEY BEGINS NOW

Your fitness journey is a personal adventure that only you can embark on. It's not about achieving someone else's standards of beauty or health; it's about becoming the best version of yourself.

You've learned about the importance of setting clear goals, creating a plan, and staying consistent. You've discovered the power of mindset and how it can influence your success. You've also been reminded that setbacks and challenges are a natural part of the journey and opportunities for growth.

Now, it's time for you to take action.

Start by setting your own fitness goals, whether they're related to weight loss, muscle gain, improved endurance, or better overall health. Create a plan that works for your lifestyle and preferences. Find ways to stay motivated and hold yourself accountable. And most importantly, embrace the journey and enjoy the process of becoming a healthier, fitter, and happier you.

Remember, your fitness journey is not just about physical transformation; it's about personal growth and self-discovery. It's about developing habits and a mindset that will serve you well for the rest of your life.

The choice is yours, and the adventure awaits.

Start by envisioning a letter to you, etched in the finest ink of your soul. Address it to the you who hungers for a healthier, fitter self, and let the words flow like a river of determination.

Paint with words the vibrant image of the person you aspire to be, not for vanity, but for the love and respect you owe your precious vessel.

Embrace the raw power that lies within you, for you are the alchemist of your own transformation. This letter, my dear friend, is the spark that ignites the flame of unwavering commitment.

It is the love song to your body, a symphony of strength and grace. Write it with the ink of your heart, sign it with the fire in your spirit, and let it be a testament to your journey towards a healthier, fitter you.

Then take action start now, and let your journey to a healthier, happier you, begin today.

Acknowledgments

In the narrative of my life, where chapters of gratitude intertwine with the raw, unfiltered moments of vulnerability, I find myself humbled by the presence of so many wonderful souls. Each one has played a unique role in shaping my journey and the words that now fill these pages.

To my cherished clients, you've not only allowed me into your lives but also into the depths of your hearts on our shared path of healing. My gratitude to you knows no bounds.

To Mr. Roques, my high school theology teacher, you ignited the spark that set my spirit on a quest for the profound search for truth.

My dear friends and colleagues, you have been the lighthouses guiding me through turbulent seas, and the winds beneath my wings when I faltered. To my fellow professionals, you have honed my skills and shaped me into the trainer I am today. To the angels disguised as life's challenges, heartaches, and crises, you bestowed upon me the gifts that define my existence.

To the sisters of my heart, my Shield Maidens, and Unstoppable Queens, your unwavering support fortified my spirit. My 5-star class act and badass coach Setema Gali you saw my potential and helped me conquer my inner demons, inspiring reps and action every single day, hence this book!

My gratitude extends to my publisher, Tammy Koelling, for taking a chance on me and my publicist, Suzi Prokell, and their dedicated teams who have transformed my words into this book that now rests in your hands.

To my family, my pillars of strength, my mother's lessons of resilience, and the wisdom of balance and moderation she instilled. My father, for your unwavering belief in goodness and a life filled with a sense of profound accomplishment, shines through me. My sister, you've been my protector and the voice of reason. My beloved Grandma Rose, your dahl soup and wisdom nourish my soul, and your laughter and courage still resonate within me.

To my soulmate and true love, my husband, B, who has nurtured my spirit, allowing me to follow my heart freely, grounding me in moments of wild dreams. To My Koa, my soul, your intuition, strength, and warrior trailblazing spirit inspire me. To Kai, your boundless heart and quick wit bring me so much joy and fill my heart with so much love. You all gifted me the privilege of motherhood, a blessing I cherish every day.

With My deepest gratitude and love,
Laine D'Souza

Author Bio

Laine D'Souza was born and raised in Hong Kong. Educated in England and earned a BA from The University of Wales. She believes all her travels make her A Child of The Universe and her home is where her family is. Laine lived in New York City where she worked as an actress, and as a certified personal trainer, and has been working in the fitness industry for the last twenty-three-plus years.

If she isn't spending time with family, you can almost always find her around her sweet Black Lab, Ninja, or her other seven equally sweet dogs writing her books. Laine can be found on her Ranch with her husband, two kids, dogs, a horse, chickens, and cows. Laine and her husband are busy building their ranch from the ground up; from building fence lines and feeding baby cows to creating RanchFit Retreats.

Laine is on a mission to help people remember who they are, and the keys to taking action towards creating daily habits to overcome debilitating self-doubt. She is also passionate about bridging the gap to help local ranchers, farmers, and artisans sell their produce, by raising people's awareness of where their food comes from and how it is produced and raised, in order to make healthier choices. Work Hard, Play Hard, Be Kind. Live Healthy, Laugh Often, Love Every Rep.

Confidence Unleashed: Be the Unstoppable Hero of Your Own Heart is Laine's first book in this series.